THE YWCA WAY
TO PHYSICAL FITNESS

THE YWCA WAY TO PHYSICAL FITNESS:
How To Make What You Have Better

---

by Evelyn Fiore

Consultant: Elaine Quinn

Based on Exercise Programs Developed by the YWCA of the City of New York

Doubleday & Company, Inc.
Garden City, New York

Library of Congress Cataloging in Publication Data

Fiore, Evelyn L., 1918–
 The YWCA way to physical fitness.

 1. Exercise for women. I. Quinn, Elaine.
II. YWCA of the City of New York. III. Title.
IV. Title: Y.W.C.A. way to physical fitness.
GV482.F55 1983b 613.7'045 82-45639
ISBN 0-385-18472-7

ISBN: 0-87469-039-0
© 1983 by Rutledge Books
Designed and Prepared for Doubleday & Company, Inc.
by Rutledge Books
All rights reserved
Doubleday & Company
245 Park Avenue
New York, N.Y. 10017

Designed by: Allan Mogel
Illustrated by: Amelia MacMahon
Interior Model: Terrylynn Smith
Cover Model: Beth Myatt

Acknowledgments

For the creation of the exercise programs in this book and for much expert input, the author is grateful to YW instructors:

Louise Charney
Elinor Coleman
Eva Dianiska
Carol Elsner
Marge Helenchild
Edna Mae Robinson
Emily Sampton
Sara Zaslow

Very special thanks are due to Madeleine Douet, the resourceful Director of the Laura Parsons Pratt Research Center of the YWCA/New York City; to Elizabeth Norris, Librarian of the YWCA National Board; to Melissa Russell, Honorary Member of the Board of Directors of the YWCA, New York City, who shared with us her vast resources of memory and experience; to Alison Fiore for much essential research assistance. Material from Dr. Sonia Weber's many works has been used here with her kind permission.

Contents

Chapter 1 1
What the YWCA Knows about Women

Chapter 2 19
What You're Working With

Chapter 3 43
Doing It

Abdomen 90 **Stretch** 62, 70, 92, 102,
Arms 62, 96   106
Buttocks 80 **Thighs** 70, 98, 100
Hips 80, 94 **Waist** 64, 66, 76,

Chapter 4 109
The Emergency Shape-Up

Chapter 5 113
The Working Back

A Last Word 164

THE YWCA WAY
TO PHYSICAL FITNESS

Chapter 1
What the YWCA Knows about Women

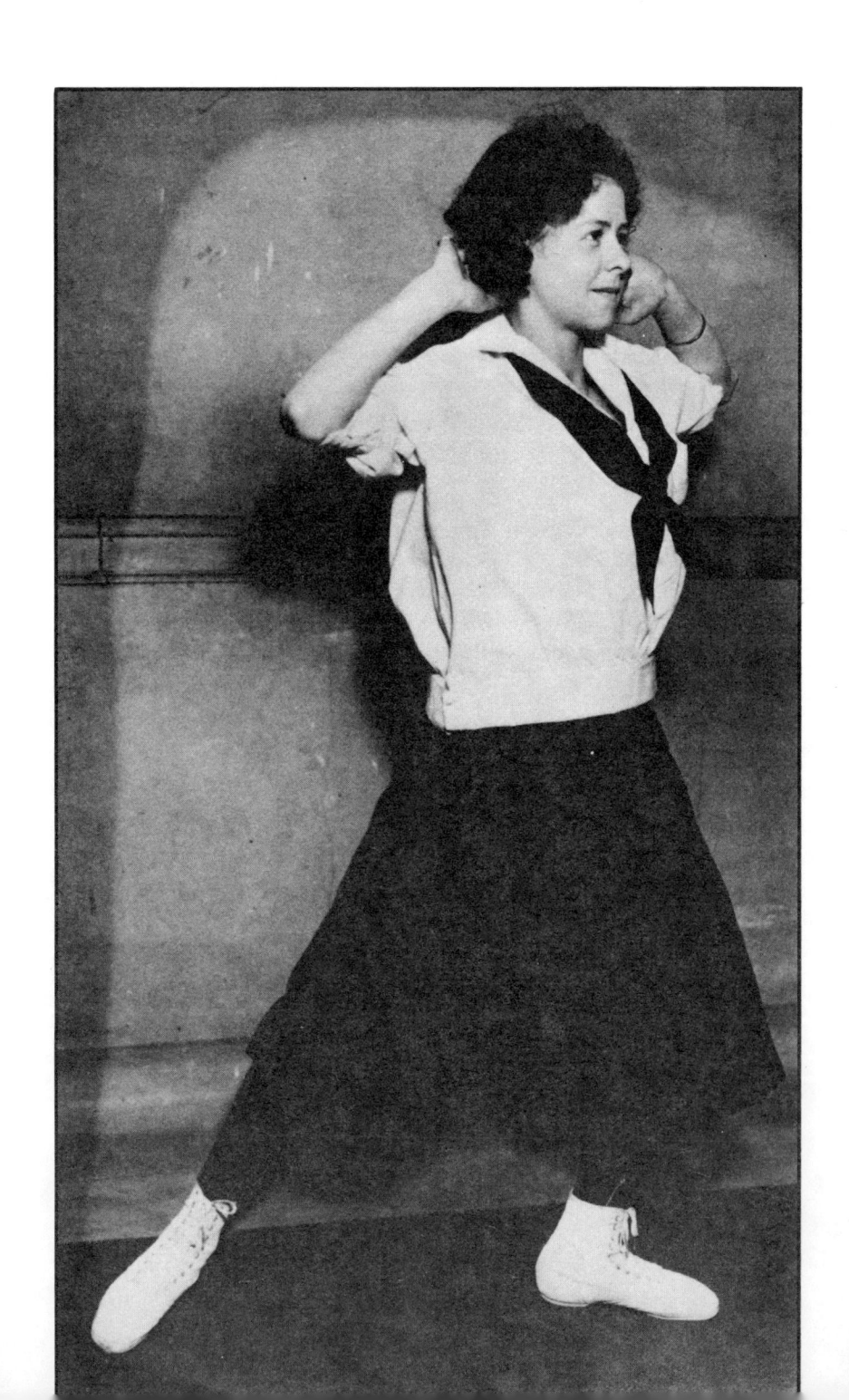

The YWCA doesn't know everything about women. Nobody ever will. Even Sigmund Freud threw up his hands and admitted that he couldn't answer "the great question: What does a woman want?"

But because the YWCA has over a hundred years of experience with women—all ages, all kinds—it can lay claim to knowing a lot. With 456 branches in the United States and hundreds more in 83 countries around the world, the YW has a pretty good idea of what women want and need at any given time.

Times change. Once it was feather curling and training on the newfangled typewriting machines. Now it's assertiveness training, investment management, living alone. Nevertheless, underneath and all along, there has been one consistent desire that never wavers. Whatever it is they're doing, women want to look their best while they're doing it.

Elizabeth Arden, Yves St. Laurent, and forty-dollar haircuts can all contribute their part toward this end. But the body they're decorating is the bottom line. If it's not limber, trim, vital—if it's not a pleasure to look at and to live in—there's nothing that can be done to the surface that will give it the eighteen-carat glow that's really what looking your best is all about.

And it won't be limber, trim, and vital unless it's exercised. Not just walked around the room a couple of times. *Exercised*.

The YW has known all about that from the start. Back when the word "body" was unacceptable in polite conversation, the YW boldly offered body-training classes to women who were bold enough to reject the conventional myth that they didn't have bodies at all—not if they were ladies. Ladies had limbs, not legs. They had the vapors then, not menstrual cramps or digestive problems.

This wasn't good enough for the YW, and it wasn't good enough for the YW's students. A first "light calisthenics" class mushroomed into physical training departments in YWCAs all across the country and indeed throughout the world, making them centers for this activity as well as for many others.

For more than 100 years of fitness fad and fashion, the YW has always focused its attention on the serious work and new developments of exercise professionals. With this background, who better than the YW to draw on its classroom wisdom to put together an exercise course for use at home?

In this book a trained and talented group of YW specialists has created such a course, drawing on all the YW's expertise and their own to construct a program you can start on now and use forever. It's sound and it's basic, designed for everyone. Nothing in it will hurt you or ask more of you than you can do. Everything in it will improve you. It will put you and your body back on good terms; there's no telling where you might go from there.

Improvement for women, hand in hand with improvement *of* women, has always been the YW's central theme. When it started out, in mid-nineteenth-century England, it was chiefly concerned with improving the moral and religious climate for young women newly employed in big cities and living for the first time on their own. But by the time the movement crossed the Atlantic, women like Lucretia Boyd, a Boston missionary, were calling for attention to other problems as well.

These self-supporting women, she told Boston's churchgoing establishment, "live in attic rooms, struggling with poverty, loneliness and isolation; neglected in sickness, helpless when out of work, and subject to chance acquaintance from the lower strata of society. Cannot something be done by benevolent ladies . . . ?"

The benevolent ladies of Boston responded by setting up

the first YWCA in the United States, in 1859.

They were not alone for long. During the next several years a scattering of YWs appeared across the country, mostly in the large industrial cities. The growth of the New York City YW was typical.

It first came together at the call of Caroline Roberts, a dynamic "benevolent lady" with years of experience in New York social work. The Ladies Christian Union, which she headed, had been quick in perceiving that if wage-earning women were to be helped, their working and living conditions had to be improved. As early as 1860, the Union started going into factories at the noon hour (their first excursion was into a hoop-skirt factory) to see firsthand how female employees were treated and to bring them a message of support.

Mrs. Roberts knew that no organization survives without a constant infusion of new blood. In January of 1870, she invited thirty-one of the Union's youngest members—girls just out of the city's most prestigious young ladies' academies—to meet in the picture gallery of her fashionable Fifth Avenue brownstone. The elegant atmosphere must have made what she had to say all the more poignant; it was the same message Lucretia Boyd had brought to Boston ten years earlier. According to the *Recollections* of Georgianna Ballard, who was one of that select group (and who would later give her name to the New York YW's renowned School of Education), "It was laid before us that there was a class of girls who were not having much in life and very little opportunity to earn anything. . . . Would we organize and do something for them?"

The New York Young Ladies Christian Association, as they first called themselves, went even further than Lucretia Boyd had gone. "To earn" became the operative words. The woman who had to earn her own living, they decided, could best be helped by being guided toward doing a better job of it. Her job opportunities, her wages, her working conditions, and her living arrangements all had to be improved.

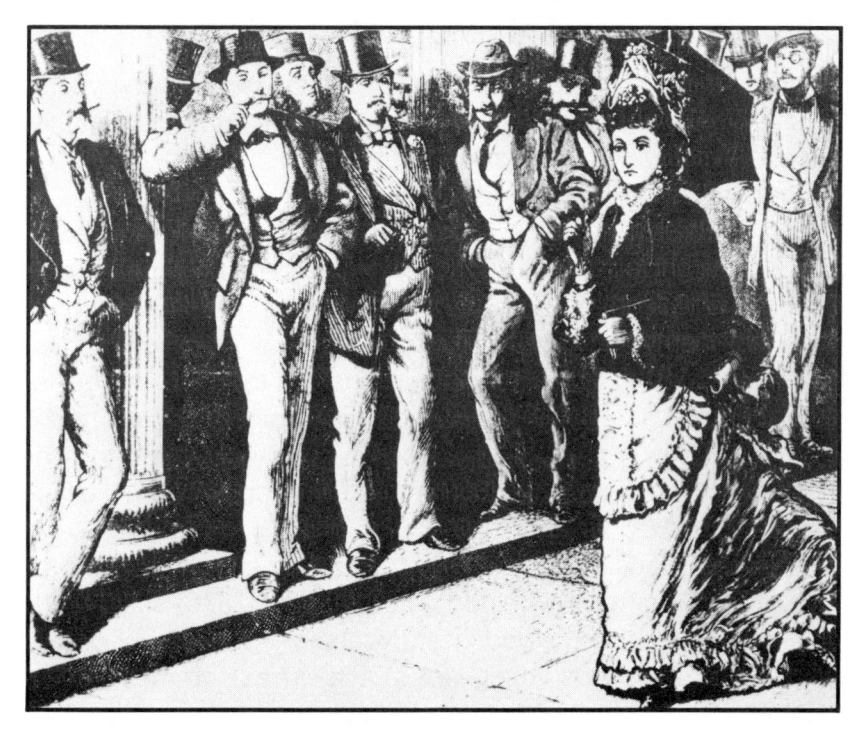

The arrogant mashers of the 1880s considered any unescorted woman fair game, making the city hazardous for working women who often had to travel alone. YWs became a welcome refuge against this nuisance..

Nobody knew for certain how many such women there were in New York at the time, nor indeed were the figures known for any of the cities in which YWs were springing up. Though the nation's census became "scientific" in 1850, it was not all that definitive. But it's safe to conclude that New York's problem was among the worst. The Association for Improving the Condition of the Poor guessed at an estimate of 70,000. Each month hundreds more came in by railroad or riverboat or horse-drawn omnibus to try their luck in the teeming city environment for which they were usually quite unprepared. They were women forced into breadwinning because their men had been killed at Shiloh or Gettysburg; women who could no longer cope on their own with family farms, or subsist on the pennies a day paid out in small-town textile mills and shoe factories.

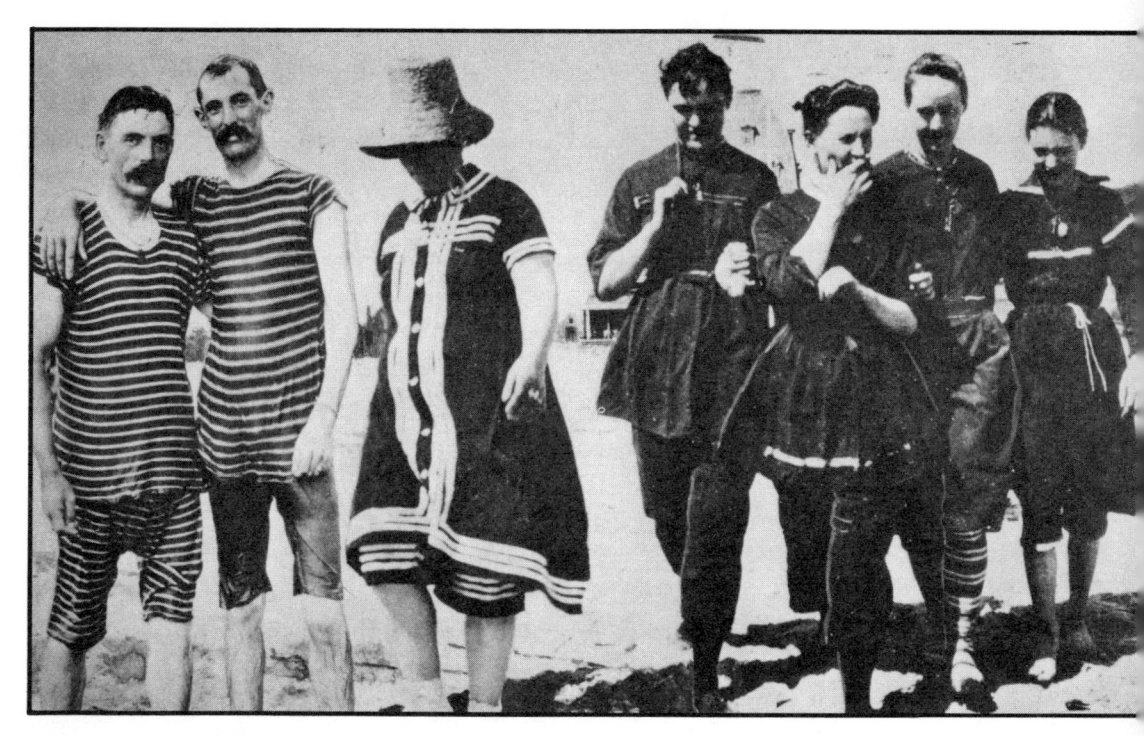

Daringly outfitted "pour le sport" in the nineties; the lady in the hat was perhaps only a sun-lover, but the trousered costumes of her friends made real swimming at least theoretically possible.

They were drawn to New York—as they were to Boston or Philadelphia or Dayton or Pittsburgh—by the hope of better wages, but their fate rarely matched those hopes. In New York most of the newcomers found their way into the needle trades, and the elite among them, those who could operate factory sewing machines, might earn up to eight dollars a week. Their working conditions were abominable. Massed like lemmings in filthy workrooms, they labored for twelve to fifteen hours a day in dust- and lint-choked air, in poor light, with toilet facilities minimal and even less care taken for other sanitary and safety needs. The early sewing machines lacked protective features we now take for granted and were a constant danger to girls made groggy by exhaustion and bad air Yet apart from the small number of women supporting themselves as teachers, these were the women at the top of the wage scale.

At the bottom was the pieceworker who worked at home. Her fifteen-hour day of shirt finishing or flower making or beadwork netted her perhaps fifty cents. Putting in six such days a week, a girl lucky enough to get steady work might manage to eat and pay her rent, but a pair of shoes or a warm coat had to be scrimped for and was not achieved nearly as often as it was needed.

Under these circumstances, illness, malnutrition, and despair defeated many a young woman's fight to remain "respectable." Lucretia Boyd had touched on the problem of "chance acquaintance from the lower strata," and there was no question that many perfectly decent young women were driven by misery into taking what was called "the easy way."

Yet tens of thousands persisted, and among them, all across the country, was a core of working women of a new breed, made up of those who dimly saw that it might not always be a calamity for a woman to be thrust out into the industrial marketplace. The thought was beginning to dawn that one day a woman might be proud of her ability to provide for herself.

Mrs. Roberts' Young Ladies went directly to the point: money. With $2603 collected from friends and families, they rented the top floor of a building on University Place and as Georgianna Ballard recorded, "hung curtains at intervals. Beyond one curtain, a Needlework Department. In another section, a shelf, and on that shelf 30 books. In another place . . . a table on which we put magazines and newspapers—the first free reading room for girls." This was monumental. Nowhere in the city was there another public library open to women. The New York Public Library wasn't fully open until 1911; until then a woman who cared to read had to have access to some private collection. With the YW founders, the emphasis on books was compulsive. They realized that reading meant the broadening of horizons, the exposure to information, and even simply new pleasure—all as essential as technical skills. Within two years those 30 books became 800,

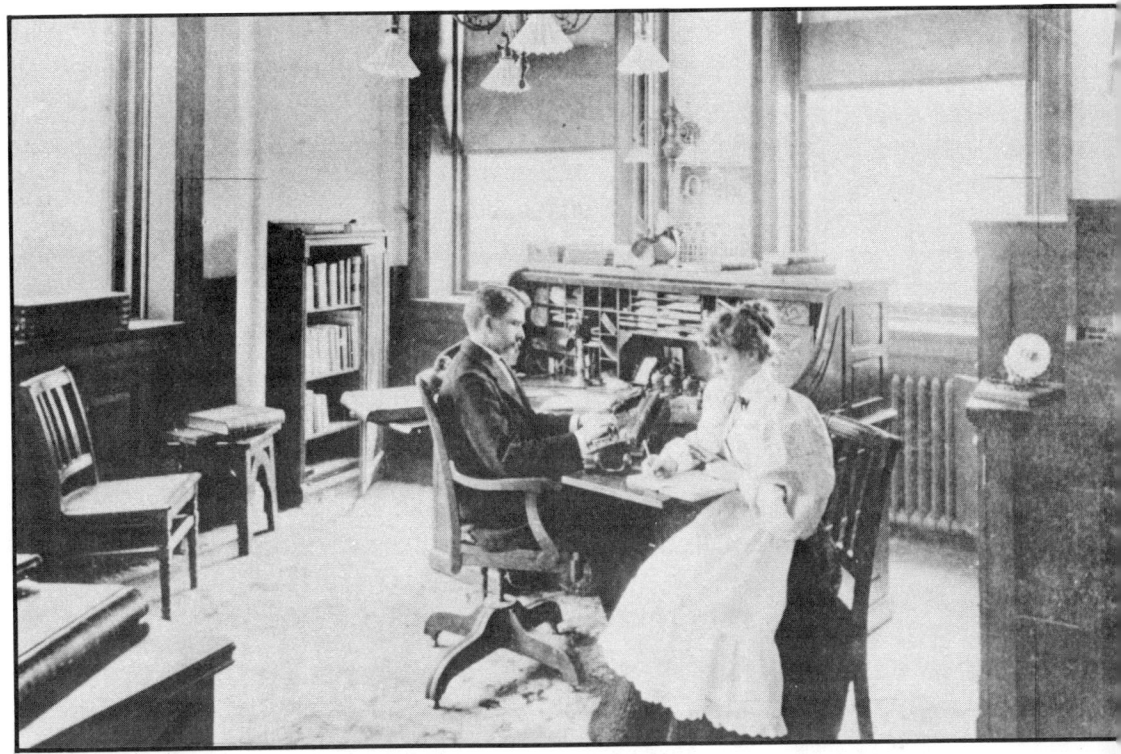

An early graduate of the YW's "phonography" classes blazes her way into the twentieth century—as does her employer, who a few years earlier would have been dictating to a male secretary.

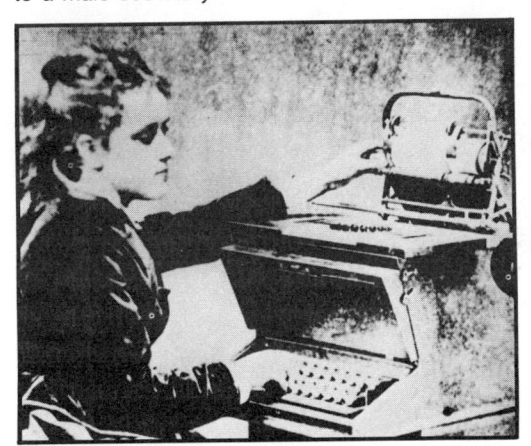

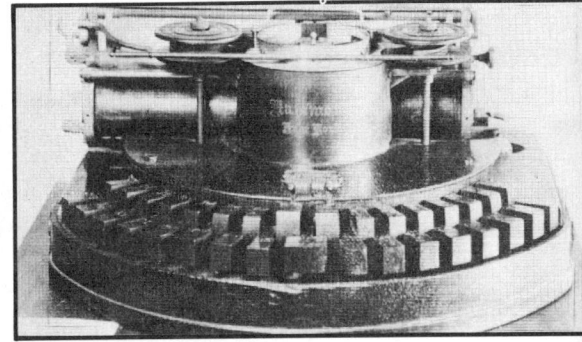

Invented in 1714, the typewriter did not become a commercial reality until 1864. Early Remingtons were cumbersome, but almost at once YW students disproved the male myth that women were too weak to handle them.

and eventually there was a YW library that could hold its own with any other in or near the city: 35,000 volumes.

With so little money to spend (all services were free at the start, and, unlike many YWs in smaller cities, managed to remain free for almost twenty years) the Young Ladies soon found they had to pitch in in unaccustomed ways. This drove off the dilettante fringe, but left a hard core of twenty-two who (again, Georgianna Ballard): ". . . fell to and cleaned floors ourselves . . . polished up gas fixtures . . . dusted and got at it with scrubbing brush. Then we organized an Evening Social with picture papers, games and puzzles, and waited for the girls to come."

It is part of YW history that for two months the games were untouched, the books unopened; nobody came. No such facilities had ever been offered before, and young women already bruised and battered by the threatening city were understandably suspicious. But finally two brave ones ventured in. The next night, they brought two more "And," one of the members wrote triumphantly, "we are on our way!"

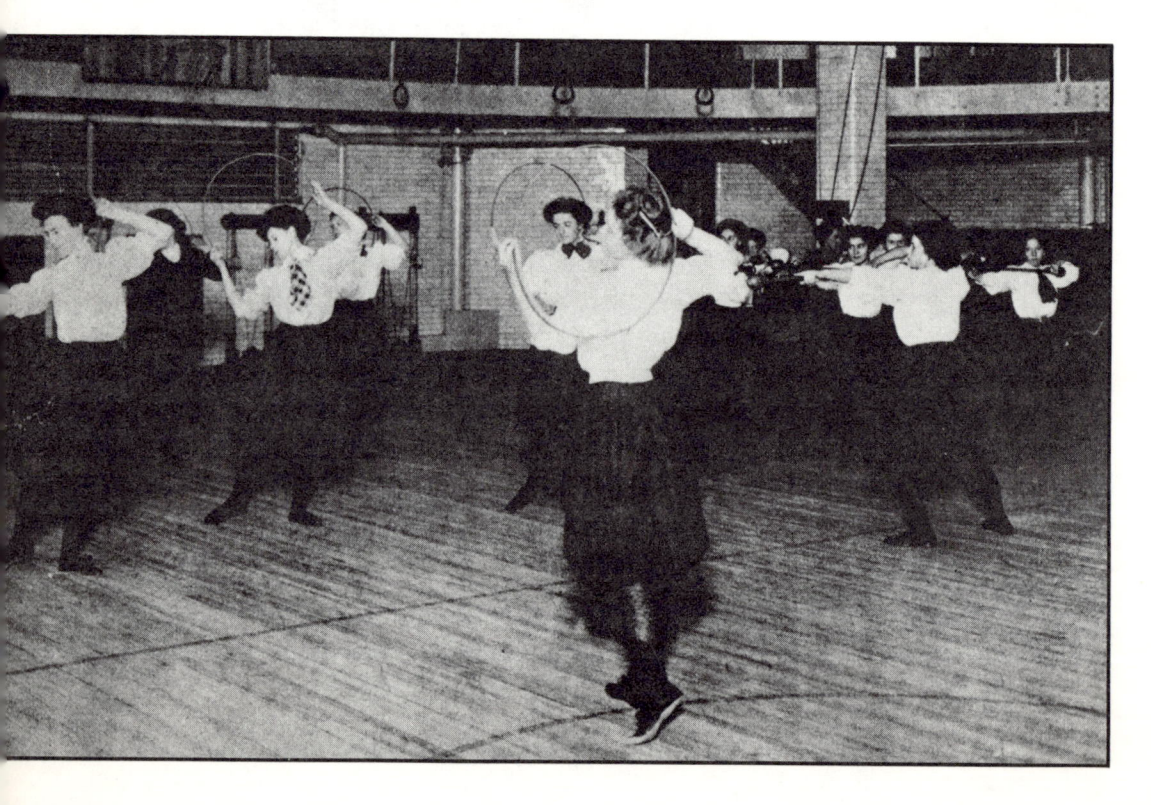

In a short time the Needlework and Dressmaking rooms were put on a businesslike basis, with a place where items made in class could be sold. There were classes in beadwork and embroidery and feather curling, an art to which the seductive fans and dramatic headgear of the period owed a lot of their graceful sweep. All across the country other YWs mirrored this kind of development. But the New York YW was facing very special urban problems, and it began to take giant steps. Shortly after its opening it established the city's first free employment bureau for women, one of the first in the nation, and by 1872 had placed 467 of the 960 who had applied—not staggering, but not bad for beginners.

Five years after their first meeting, New York knew that the Young Ladies Christian Association was around to stay. They were set up in much larger quarters—the result of their increasing adeptness at raising money—and thousands of girls each year used their facilities. They had a serious place in the life of the city, and they marked it in a significant way. They changed their name to the Young *Women's* Christian Association. "Woman," they felt, conveyed a more mature, responsible image than "lady," and better underlined that they were no longer amateurs, but professionals in their chosen work. And five years after that, in 1880, they organized a new activity which in effect put their employment program over the top. They set up courses in stenography (then known as phonography) and typewriting.

This was not as simple as saying, "We'll do it." Secretarial work was a male preserve. In the conventional wisdom of the time, women's brains were not considered up to the demands of stenography. And how could frail females imagine that they could manipulate cumbersome typewriting machines, even the newly practical Remingtons, without doing themselves bodily harm?

Working five days a week for six months, the stenography students showed themselves so adept that at graduation almost all were snapped up. Prospects for the "typewriters" (these were the women, not the machines) were at first less promising. Prejudice was deep against females trying to invade still another male preserve. But the YW worked out a brilliant bit of salesmanship: it invited potential employers to come in and observe their class at work. That demonstration was all it took. The graduates of that class all walked out into jobs that paid more than any of them had ever hoped to earn. By the end of 1885, the YW employment bureau had placed 12,454 of its 18,729 registrants, a huge upsurge that was due to its new army of typists and stenographers. So pay and prospects were inching upward. All over the country YWs were increasingly alert to the job-connected needs not only of their own members but of all young women. Noontime visits to factories, when the girls were on their own time and no employer could object, became a regular YW habit. In Pittsburgh YW women talked to girls in cigar factories and bakeries; in Kalamazoo they went to paper mills, and in South Carolina to cotton mills; the Dayton, Ohio, National Cash Register plant could count on its "Busy Girls' Half Hour" every Monday noontime, when the local YW brought some of its activities to girls who could otherwise not get to them. News about women's progress and problems was thus spread among women who had few other ways of obtaining it.

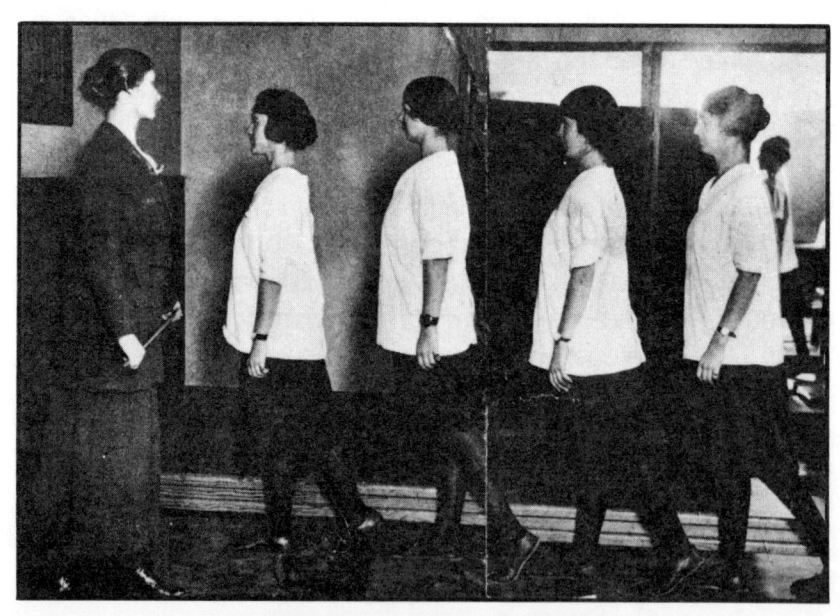

Circa 1914; drills were still semi-military, but uniforms were making progress. Bloomers, though still capacious, were lighter than before, and short-sleeved middies made movement much freer.

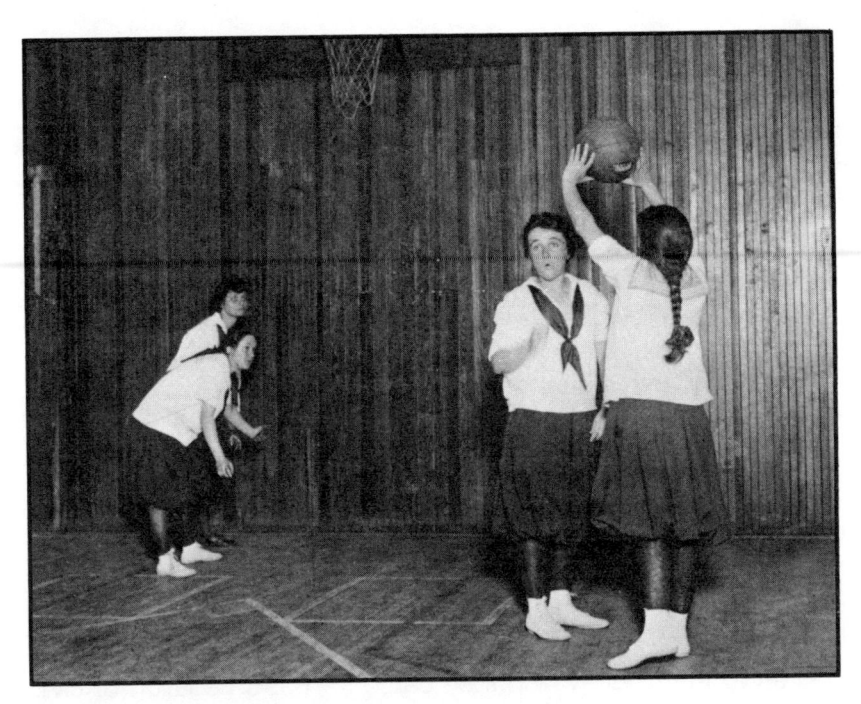

Men played basketball for years before it was available to women. In the 1920s YWs encouraged not only the game but the new idea that women, given the chance, made perfectly good team players.

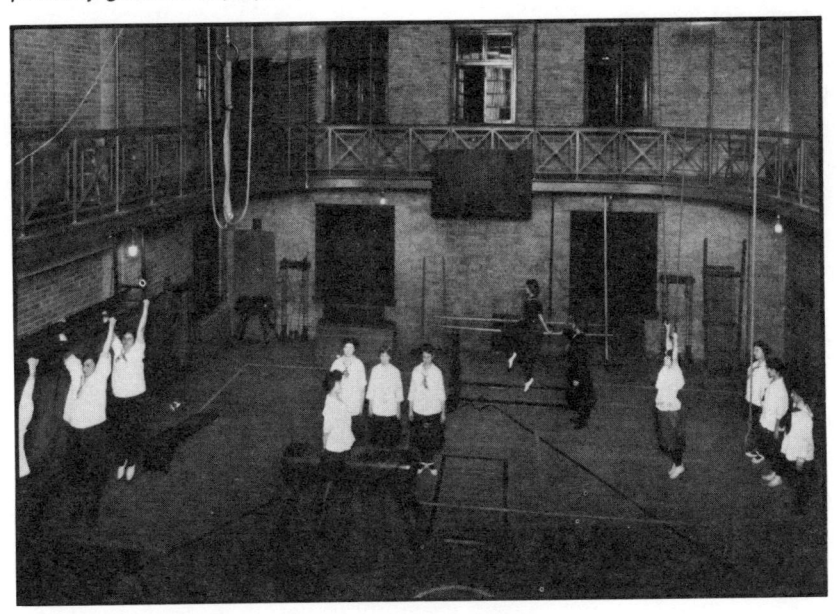

The "new" New York YW gym, circa 1922: increasingly adept, young women could really work out on this up-to-date and well constructed equipment. Some of it remained in use until fairly recent years.

Reaching out in this way toward women, YWs all over the country quickly demonstrated that they meant *all* women—a remarkable sensitivity to racial problems that were barely coming to the surface. In 1882 the Pittsburgh branch opened a home for Negro orphans. A few years later the first all-black YW was set up in Dayton, Ohio. By 1899, American Indian women had their own branch at Haworth Institute in Oklahoma, and as more black and Indian student associations formed at other colleges they were welcomed into the YW orbit. Through the years the YW's interracial programs strengthened and expanded, always tending toward equality and integration. In the 1930s black members were moving into leadership positions, and the organization was making itself heard in thorny racist situations: lynchings, mob violence against blacks, the infamous Scottsboro case in Alabama. In 1942, while the United States was still at war, the YW spoke out courageously against the internment of Japanese-Americans in this country—an action widely publicized nowadays but largely ignored at the time—which they called "a basic negation of civil liberties and one of the most flagrant cases of color discrimination" in our history. In 1946, the YWCA became the first national organization to officially desegregate, with the issuance of its Interracial Charter.

In April of 1970, the National Board of the YWCA codified its point of view on discrimination into a principle it calls the "One Imperative: to eliminate racism wherever it exists and by any means necessary." This statement sums up how the organization has always operated, and how it means to keep operating as long as these problems persist.

Its other principle, clear from the start, was that it must try to guide women toward a better total life, not just a better working life. As the young founders educated themselves about sweatshops and slum living, they realized that as essential as it was to have a job, it was equally essential that a young woman stay healthy while she was doing it. Most of the jobs women did kept them indoors, physically constrained; even if not all were as damaging as the sweatshop jobs, few of them did a worker's physical and mental well-being much good.

In the 1870s the Boston YW pioneered a somewhat tentative exercise class, not certain if the girls would take to it or indeed if their fragile physiques could stand it. Very shortly they had their answer, and in 1887 the New York YW followed with its first class in physical culture. Young women who worked all day at "cramped and confining toil" would now have at least a once-a-week chance to stretch, limber up, and change the pace of their breathing.

Games and regular periods of exercise were already standard at most of the men's colleges and many of the women's, their value recognized in toning up both mental and physical performance. But women who scurried to work along dirty city streets, tussled for hours with machines or crouched over desks, and then returned to living quarters where there was no room to swing a cat or even to keep one, had few opportunities to leap for volley balls or try the smart new game of lawn tennis. There were hardly any places where they could safely take a brisk walk in fresh air.

Boston need not have worried about its experimental class. A few short years later the fifth floor of the Boston YW building was entirely given over to physical education. The New York class too was inundated and rapidly became one of the New York YW's most popular offerings. Five other YWs followed, with similar classes in "light calisthenics to piano accompaniment." As new branches came into the Association movement, or as established YWs rebuilt and expanded, gymnasiums were planned into their facilities. YWs came to be synonymous with giving high priority to the sound body as well as the sound mind.

The exercises themselves, in those trailblazing days, were not very ambitious. Apart from the still-new college programs there was little tradition to draw on in training women's bodies, since for a few hundred years good form had decreed that from the neck down they were, under their clothes, invisible. The first

YW "light calisthenics" students worked out on lunging, bending, and stretching movements derived from male sports like fencing. Some material was adapted from drills used in military academies. This meant a good deal of eyes-right lining up and marching in rigid formation, plus snappy routines with wands, dumbbells, and Indian clubs. After a while hoops were added, making for a less military effect, but like the other equipment lending themselves well to precision drills. The saving grace was that all this was "performed to piano accompaniment." Some of the working women were no more than fifteen; they must have relished the chance to move around to what we can only hope was lively music, no matter what moves they were instructed to make.

In fact they got so good at their wand and hoop drills that they were soon giving demonstrations for invited audiences to great applause. The guests were often good contributors, and treasuries tended to swell nicely after a performance because the girls were marvelous advertisements for the Association's work. One New York reporter described seeing them arrive for a demonstration looking pinched and weary from their day's labors. "Afterward," he wrote, "they left with rosy cheeks, rested limbs, and erect shoulders." What better proof that the YW was offering a desperately needed activity!

Nevertheless, there were plenty of diehards around who paled at the notion of females exerting themselves in even the mildest gymnastics. And the exercise outfits, which occasionally revealed an ankle or an inch of calf—a scandal! When girls at the University of Nebraska put on gym clothes for the first time, there was chaos. "Most of the girls were so shy," the school officials were told, "that they sank down on the gymnasium floor, huddling together and almost in tears." An extreme reaction, since if their uniform was anything like the one required at Vassar, it consisted of a high-necked, long-sleeved, ankle-length dress of gray flannel, with long bloomers under the skirt.

Considering the restrictions imposed by such outfits, whatever the girls managed to do was remarkable. Even without corsets—and while in theory no lady removed hers until she was ready for bed, nobody could have survived ten minutes of gym work wearing one—free and vigorous movement must have been almost impossible. But women were seeing the future. The whole country was increasingly sports-conscious. Tennis and golf clubs arose for those who could afford them. There was spreading excitement about spectator sports. There were health buffs like the rising young politician Teddy Roosevelt, who was widely known to have built his weak physique into a robust macho image with training and exercise.

With all this going on, could exposed female ankles be far behind? In England a dashing young aristocrat turned up on the hunting field in an unheard-of calf-length riding skirt. Soon afterward an American manufacturer was advertising a gymnasium costume—in itself proof of the growing market—showing a calf-length tunic. Under the tunic, true enough, were long trousers, but the signposts were up. In the early 1900s popular women's magazines illustrated loose waists and divided skirts as "active sports costumes" for middle-class women to make from patterns.

There was no turning back. Having found out what brisk moving around could do for their bodies, their nervous systems, and their complexions, women were not about to be pushed back into passivity. And since all this moving around couldn't be done in whalebone and bustles, they were damning the torpedoes, even those from ultra-conservative critics, and charging full steam ahead.

At the YWs, middie blouses grew shorter. Sleeves were rolled up, then chopped off; the girls got used to showing some skin. Bloomers too were shortened, though well down toward World War I the regulation still decreed that they contain no less than seven yards of serge, a formidable weight; and legs were still covered with dark stockings. It's interesting that while today's second-skin leotards are a quantum leap away from those thick blouses and bloomers, legs are still covered, though now it's by tights or pantyhose, and no longer for modesty but to avoid chilled muscles.

Even without the fashion factor, costumes would inevitably

have been trimmed and trimmed again as exercises became more vigorous and demanding. Programs expanded. A few colleges set up new departments giving degrees in physical education, and as graduates trickled out they were quickly absorbed into schools and camps, as well as YMs and YWs.

In 1916, the coming of Dr. Helen McKinstry to what was by then the New York YW's growing Department of Physical Culture upgraded their program into a new professionalism. A perfectionist with a strong personal philosophy of what physical training was all about, she held the YW's students to standards of deportment, dress, and achievement that they weren't always eager to go along with. The new jazz beat that the girls would have liked for their workouts had to fight its way in against Dr. McKinstry's more sedate preferences. Nor did bobbed hair go down well with her; she wanted the girls to keep their hair long and secure it under nets for classes. Rebelling and grumbling, the students nevertheless kept coming. They knew they were getting outstanding training. In fact Dr. McKinstry took the program through the stratosphere. Transforming one group of classes into a training program for teachers of physical education, she eventually went with it, as administrator, when the YW sold it to Russell Sage College in Troy, N.Y.

The New York YW's present Department of Health, Physical Education and Recreation (HPER) grows out of this legacy of hard work and high standards. Its program reflects what is available at most YWCAs.

More than 6,000 women went through the New York YW's exercise classes last year. Purely under the law of averages they have to represent every size, shape, and degree of strength and coordination possible, and somewhere in there are at least a few like you. The teachers who develop programs for this vast variety of individuals, and who bring their students along into greatly improved physical tone, looks, and general well-being, have worked out the program in this book. They've considered the fact that you will not be working with an instructor, and they've eliminated anything difficult, dangerous, or nonproductive. Every movement they're counseling you to make is significant if your physical condition has been on your mind.

If you're serious about getting yourself into shape, you won't get better help than you'll find here.

Chapter 2
What You're Working With

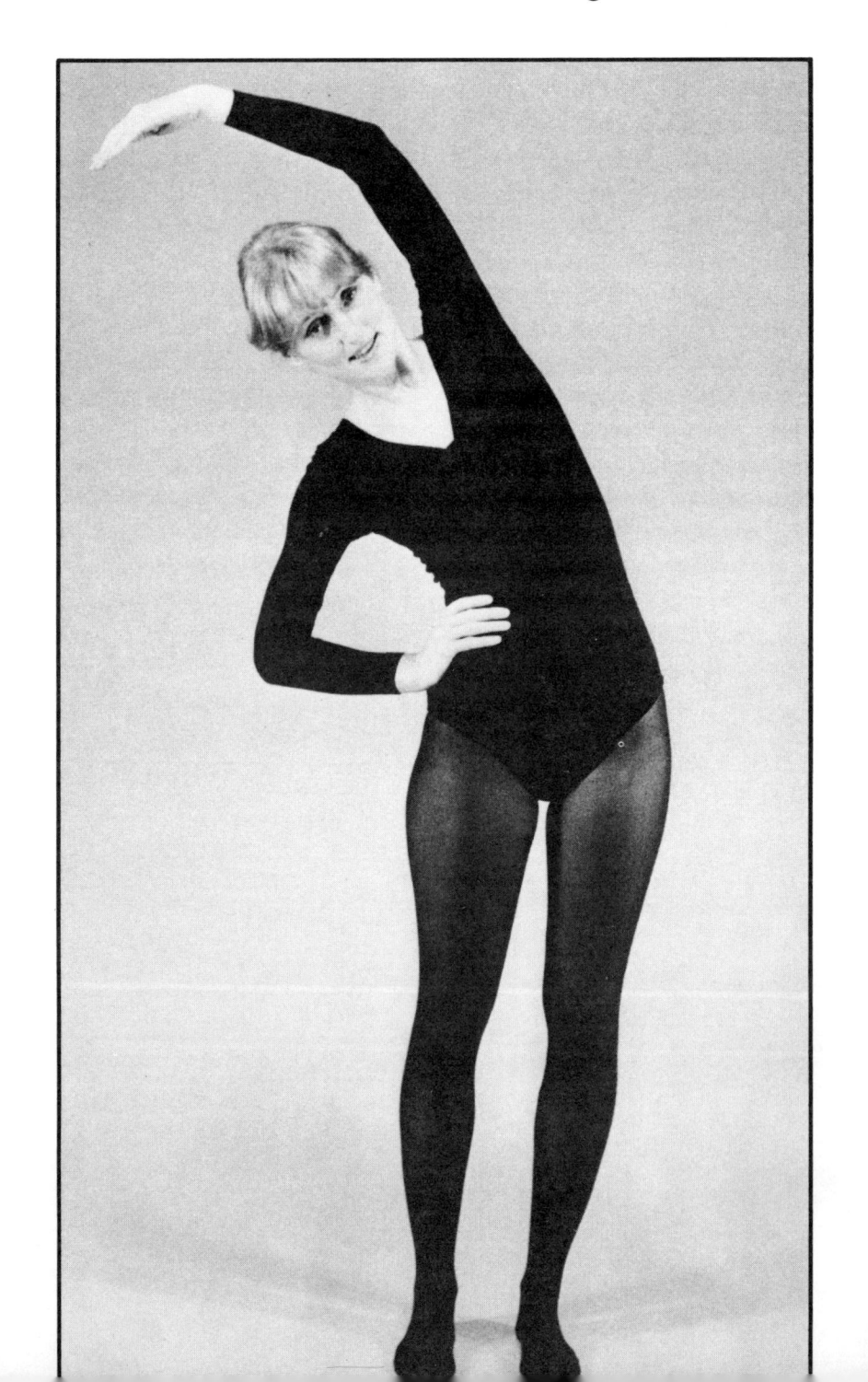

I f you've got it, keep it. That's part of the message of this book. If you're past eighteen and you're happy with the way you look and function, congratulations. But don't lean too complacently on what was probably genetic good fortune. It's a wise woman who, recognizing that from here on it's uphill every year, sets up her defenses early. Form an exercise habit when you're young and don't need repair work: that's the ideal way. Usually you'll get hooked on it, and you'll keep it working for you.

However, here you are, and you *haven't* got it anymore—not the way you'd like it, anyway. You bulge and puff, maybe more than a bit. You don't own a skirt you can fasten without holding your breath; there's no zipper in your wardrobe that slides up to a perfect finish. Maybe you were out of shape before you knew you were out of shape, before it showed. By the time you're facing trouble in your mirror, a lot of slippage and softening up has already gone on under the skin. That can happen, as it were, behind your back, because your body is one of the most incredibly complicated mechanisms known to man—large areas of it are in fact not fully known, because their subtleties have so far eluded our most sophisticated research.

Luckily, we know that barring illness or accident, you can have a lot of control over your complex body network. You can feed it properly, see that it gets enough rest, and keep it exercised so that it functions at maximum efficiency. Feeding and resting come almost automatically; at least we know when we're ignoring the signals. We know well enough when we're hungry, though we don't always know when to stop eating. And when our eyes close and our minds drift there's no doubt we need rest.

But exercise starvation can be more easily concealed or disguised. Tiring easily? We're bored with our jobs. Fretful and snappish? Overwork, or a run-in with a traffic cop. Really extreme fatigue? Strange aches? We're catching something. Maybe. But these symptoms may really be telegraphing underused muscles. The effects are not always superficial and transitory. Some years ago Dr. Hans Kraus and Dr. Wilhelm Raab coined the term "hypokinetic disease" for a long list of genuine illnesses they believe arise from muscular neglect.

You only have to think about it for a minute to realize that the way most of us live promotes this underuse. We don't need to climb trees for food, run from hungry tigers, or—until lately—chop wood for fuel unless we choose to. All of that activity kept the human body in better shape in days gone by. The girls in those early YW classes probably walked to work to save carfare, climbed up and down stairs many times a day, lugged buckets of laundry and coal, did their washing and ironing by hand, and met a hundred other physical demands we now cope with by flicking switches. Yet even they knew they needed exercise, and gave up precious evening leisure for it as soon as somebody gave them the chance.

Stress and tension hadn't yet become household words, but those women must have realized that after their classes they felt "unwound" and relaxed, and in spite of the output of energy they were less tired than when they entered the gym. They may have felt less depressed; exercise will do that for you too. Probably they noticed that it became easier to push those heavy typewriter carriages and run those foot-powered sewing machines for hours at a time. The strength and tone of their muscles were being improved by exercise.

This in turn affected their looks—as it will yours. In their day vanity was a cardinal sin, so perhaps they tried not to think too much about those "rosy cheeks" and gratifyingly slender waists. But in the 1980s you're free to put the cosmetic effects of exercise above all the other good things it will do for you if that's what it takes to get you moving.

It's the word "moving" that's crucial. The body was made to move, not to spend most of every day sitting, riding, and constricted, getting its major workout waiting on lines at the supermarket or running across the street against traffic. If it isn't triggered into movement reasonably often, for a reasonable length of time, at a stimulating pace, the body bogs down. The skeleton starts to lose the constant battle it must wage against the pull of gravity, and it sags—enter back problems, leg problems, headaches. Circulation is sluggish: the skin and eyes are dull; the heart function isn't what it should be; the brain is shortchanged of the oxygen it needs for its best performance. As for the muscles, they suffer most. Some stretch. Some tighten up and lose their resilience. Fatty deposits accumulate that are far harder to get rid of than to prevent. As the whole maltreated mechanism slows down, wastes that should be quickly and regularly thrown off cannot be handled efficiently and tend to accumulate—enter constipation, fatigue, and a good percentage of Hamlet's "thousand natural shocks that flesh is heir to."

This body, to speak moderately, is not physically fit, a condition that the President's Council on Physical Fitness describes as having "the ability to carry out daily tasks with vigor and alertness, and with ample energy to enjoy leisure and to meet unforeseen emergencies." Since most of our unforeseen emergencies don't involve fighting forest fires or pulling fallen oaks off trapped victims, we can scrape through, most of the time, without full awareness that what we think of as vigor and alertness are really pale versions of what they could be. Yet consider, even if our emergencies aren't always dramatic, there's no lifestyle these days that guarantees there will be none. Vast electrical systems fail and city folk with unpracticed legs have to somehow get up to the tenth floor. Anyone may have to fight off a mugger any day of his life, and that's becoming run-of-the-mill even for suburbanites. You may have to chase a speedy five-year-old who's determined to get where you've told him he can't go, and not be too wiped out to scold him when you do catch him. All emergencies call for a sudden, unexpected spurt of energy and muscular response. We should be able to exert ourselves when necessary. For a body in good shape, it's no problem.

The point of this book is that exercise will help you get into this kind of shape. You could go from here directly to the exercises themselves, but trust the YW's experience—you'll get far more out of them if you pause now to become familiar with your raw materials, the parts of your body you'll be working with. We're not talking about a course in physiology. All we need here is a stringently simplified, bottom-line view—or review, since a lot of this background was in the hygiene and biology classes we had back in school—of what our skeleton and muscles do in and for our bodies.

The time you spend on the next few pages will pay off in benefits. The YW instructors, if they could, would ask all their students to bone up (no pun intended) on this material before entering a class. Students appear to get more out of each exercise when they're aware of what muscles are being set in motion. When you know where the deltoids are and what they're for, you can see in your mind's eye what happens to them, and to other associated muscles, when you raise your arms. This way you get a better kinesthetic (muscle sense) feel for what's going on as you exercise. With an enhanced awareness of muscle movement and sensation, you almost subconsciously make a much more deliberate, strenuous effort to get all the stretch and reach you can out of even a simple motion.

The Skeleton

Before we deal with the muscles, let's pause (see page 23) at the skeleton, because these bones describe certain limits as to what you can hope to accomplish.

Your skeleton is the foundation for your size and structure, and to some extent for your shape and proportions. Usually it

ADULT SKELETON

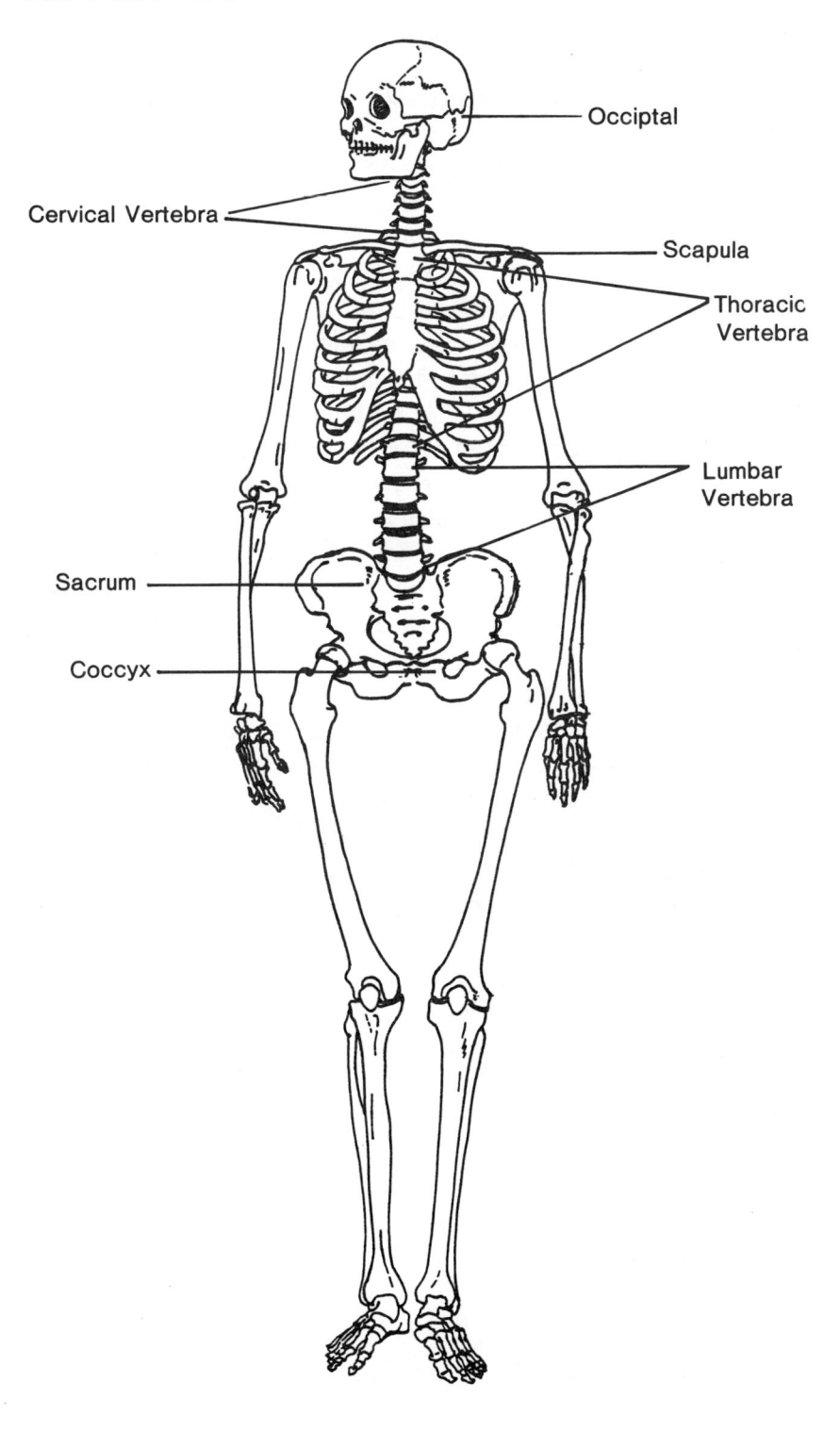

- Occiptal
- Cervical Vertebra
- Scapula
- Thoracic Vertebra
- Lumbar Vertebra
- Sacrum
- Coccyx

contains 206 bones, though very occasionally an oddity occurs, like an individual with 13 ribs to a side instead of the normal 12. Between individuals the bones vary in length and thickness. But in a single skeleton they are so precisely proportioned to one another that from a single prehistoric leg bone anthropologists can confidently construct entire skeletons of creatures they have never seen. In criminal medicine, there are sculptors who specialize in working on otherwise unidentifiable skulls, using the bones as guides in building up what usually turn out to be amazingly accurate likenesses of the individual as he was in life.

On its own, the skeleton is completely immobile. It can move only as the muscles attached to it dictate. But that doesn't mean it just stands there. It's responsible for several life-supporting functions. It protects bone marrow in which red blood cells are formed, and supplies the body with phosphorus, calcium, and other essential elements. It also stores protein on which the body can draw at need.

In one sense, however, it does just stand there. Now that you're adult, your skeleton has done all the growing and changing for which it was genetically programmed. It has benefited as much as it's going to from the balanced diet and vitamin supplements and all-round good health advice that parents and teachers and doctors have been forcing on you all during your developing years. Speaking from an exercise viewpoint, there's not much you can do about your particular collection of bones except learn to hold and move it correctly.

In other words, what you've got is what you must live with. If your antecedents bequeathed you a swanlike neck, a long-boned torso, a narrow pelvic girdle, and long leg bones, you need the sense and discipline to keep all that from disappearing under layers of fat and out-of-shape muscle.

But suppose you had a different legacy, and you've come up with shorter, thicker bones and a rib cage that ends two inches or so above the top of the pelvic girdle. These can be hard lines, but only if you let them thicken and grow sloppy. You can learn to keep them taut and trim by learning how to stand up properly (page 62). (While you're thinking about page 62, go and look in the mirror again. You'll probably see a slight change already, just in the way you're carrying yourself. That's not even posture. It's attitude. Thinking of yourself as improvable is an important first step.)

Long or short, the bones are either joined together immovably, as in the skull, or linked together with tissues, called ligaments, at points of contact called joints. There are several different kinds of joints in the body, all marvelously engineered for their place and purpose. For example, at the knee, which is called upon for powerful leverage, is the body's largest joint, a condylar, which looks something like the head of a judge's gavel fitted into a miniature trough. While built for strength, it permits only limited movement. The knee can only bend and extend (straighten); if it does anything else, it's because something's gone wrong. On the other hand, ball-and-socket joints like those of the shoulder and hip give an enormously wide range of movement.

To make articulation smooth and painless, all movable joints are linked with membranes lubricated by a secretion called synovial fluid. If for some internal reason the supply is not adequate, pain and damage can result from the friction. This is not a common problem; far more common is an overproduction of fluid caused by injury or strain. Collecting in the joint, this excess fluid causes the painful inflammation we call bursitis, housemaid's knee, or tennis elbow.

Concentrate a little on our drawing of the spine. It's important; everything depends on it and from it, in the actual sense that it holds everything upright. It bears this load without being solid, or even in a strict sense straight. It does start out fairly straight at birth, but as body weight gradually increases, the 33 vertebrae that compose the spinal column shift slightly at the neck and lower back. The slight curves thus created help to carry weight and absorb shock that might otherwise cause injury. But when we fall into bad posture habits so that the curves become exaggerated, we invite other sorts of injury.

Threaded through the vertebrae is the spinal cord, protected by the bones themselves and also by spinal fluid and sheathings of tissue. Of the 31 pairs of nerves that go from this vital message center to the brain, about half are the motor nerves that convey the brain's orders to the muscles and are thus responsible for movement.

Considering how marvelously the spine is designed and protected, we must be doing something very wrong to suffer as many back problems as we do. A lot of back trouble begins with the spinal discs, cushions of cartilage filled with gelatinous material that rest between the vertebrae and prevent them from grinding against one another. Discs unfortunately can be, and often are, injured in ways that reduce or entirely destroy their cushioning ability. Worse, and more difficult to diagnose, are the sometimes unfelt injuries that rupture the disc's envelope so that the material inside escapes. This can eventually press on an adjacent nerve and cause severe pain.

Some back problems, however, are directly traceable to weakness somewhere among the 400 muscles that support the spine. Posture, again, is the most common culprit. We sink into too-low, oversoft chairs, crouching for hours with our backs bent into half-hoops, throwing strain on areas never meant to bear it. Instead of using our knees for leverage, we bend from the waist to pick up a heavy load, forcing the relatively weak small of the back to do work it cannot cope with. Over and over, when you get to the exercises, you will see that we emphasize the correct handling of this lumbar area. It should never be permitted to sway forward. It suffers already from extra demands made on it when the abdominal muscles are not doing 100 percent of their own job, which unhappily is the case with most of us, especially as we get older.

Because the back is such a vulnerable area, and because so many people develop problems with it, the YW offers a special Back Care program, developed by orthopedic specialists, which has had a remarkable success rate. See page 113 for a version of it that you can do on your own.

The Muscles

After dealing with the intractable skeleton, with its like-me-or-lump-me attitude, it's encouraging to investigate an area over which we do have some control: our muscles. We possess two kinds of muscles, the voluntary, or skeletal; and the involuntary. Through them we can do a great deal about the way we look outside and something about what goes on inside as well.

The activities inside your body are principally controlled by the *involuntary* muscles, which carry out some of the body's most vital activities. They are the smooth muscles of the stomach and intestines and other organs, and the minute ones that line the veins and arteries. They're involuntary, obviously, because basically they do their work entirely on their own. It's possible that one day science may be able to teach us how to exercise a degree of control over them, but as of now the only way we can affect them is through the body's general condition. If our body is in top shape, these muscles reflect it and carry out their part of the job with maximum efficiency. Unfortunately, poor condition is reflected too. Our emotions affect them (think what happens to your digestion when you're frightened or upset), though we have a great deal yet to learn about the actual mechanisms by which this happens.

The most important of these involuntary organs is, of course, the heart—or rather the cardiac muscle in the wall of the heart. Normally, this powerful muscle pumps 3200 gallons of blood through the system each day, carrying digested nutrients and oxygen without which body cells cannot live. This blood makes a return trip to the heart, bearing away carbon dioxide and other wastes, which then must be filtered through the lung capillaries before the purified blood is once again pumped through the body.

The heart has all the strength it needs to pump blood out. But for the return trip it must call on all kinds of help from muscles disposed throughout the body. For example, the movement of your diaphragm as you breathe helps because it compresses the

SKELETAL MUSCLES (Frontal View)

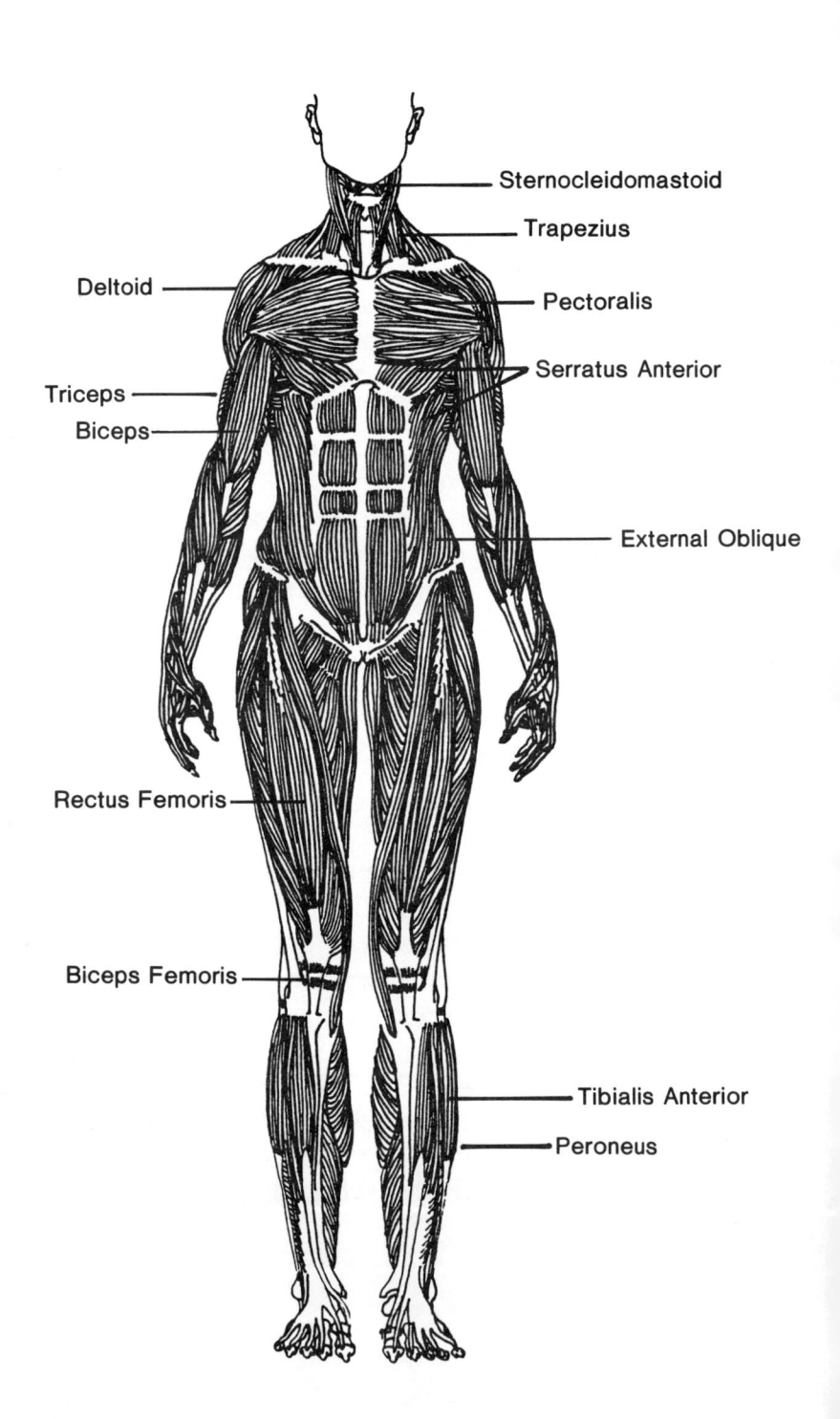

SKELETAL MUSCLES (Dorsal View)

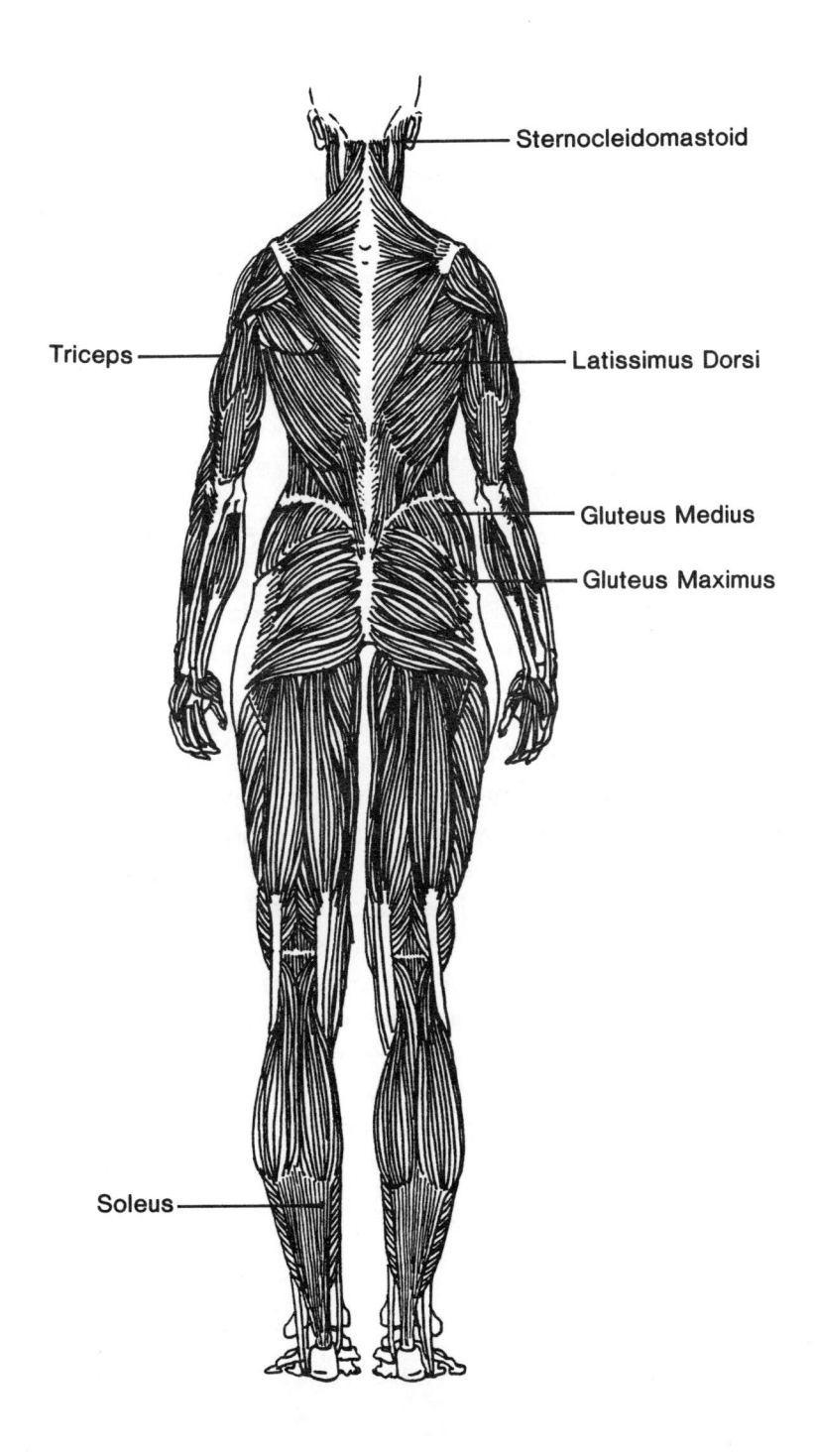

- Sternocleidomastoid
- Triceps
- Latissimus Dorsi
- Gluteus Medius
- Gluteus Maximus
- Soleus

abdominal cavity, increasing the pressure that stimulates the pumping activity of the muscles there. Surprisingly, even the muscles in the limbs help, acting as pumps to return the blood to the heart.

Although ordinary movement and muscle tone are generally sufficient for the blood's round trip, any improvement in their operation tones up not only circulation and respiration, but other functions as well, like digestion and excretion. This travel track of the blood is your circulo-respiratory system, and many experts consider it the most important single factor in what might be called your physical fitness profile. There is much current research to show that when circulo-respiratory power and endurance are high, we are better protected against heart attacks and a host of lesser problems as well.

This explains the relatively recent explosion of interest in aerobic exercise, which—to oversimplify—aims at stepping up the heartbeat and rate of respiration at a gradual and monitored pace to achieve a safe and efficient maximum. The premise is that gradually stimulating the heart and lungs to their best performance allows them to perform at a far better level during our ordinary activities. Working better, these organs provide a team that requires less effort to produce better circulation of the blood through the system. The end product is that an individual with a good circulo-respiratory function accomplishes this with a heart that actually requires fewer beats to the minute. Intensive aerobic activity can actually increase the size of the heart. It was once believed that the enlarged hearts of athletes were unhealthy by-products of their sustained and intensive exertions. But scientific opinion changes as new evidence comes in. The larger heart is now considered to be a healthier, more effective organ.

The YW offers many classes in aerobic exercise and dance, but we don't suggest such activities here because they're not something the novice should plunge into at home on her own. If you're interested, take a well-supervised class to start. It will teach you what you must know, which is What, How Much, and How

Fast makes sense for you. Most important, it will teach you how to take and keep track of your own heart and pulse rates so that you'll know what you're doing—an absolute essential with aerobic activity.

However, you can do yourself plenty of aerobic good on your own. Swimming, walking fast, even dancing are considered useful activities. In fact any movements that employ large muscle groups in fairly rapid, continuous effort are beneficial. That kind of aerobic stimulation is open to you. And you'll find that if you combine it with our exercise program, you'll perform better at both activities and increase not only the benefits but the pleasure you get from each of them.

The *voluntary* muscles are our most urgent concern, not only because they are to a large extent under our control but because they are chiefly what an exercise program is all about. It's the shape, size, tone, and general condition of these muscles that sculpt the figures we show the world; they are far more important to this final effect than are the bones to which they are attached.

Essentially these muscles (usually striated, as distinct from the smooth involuntary group) are ropes, sometimes quite broad, composed of masses of thin fibers sheathed in tissue and attached to the bones they control by tough bands of tissue called tendons. There are more than 200 pairs of them, and it is through about 75 of these pairs that we walk, sit, turn, lift, and make all the other voluntary body movements.

These muscles are activated by impulses that travel down from the brain along nerve fibers; at the junction of two nerve fibers (called a synapse), the impulse triggers the production of a chemical substance (acetylcholine) that jumps the synapse and provokes a contraction of the muscle fibers.

Almost all muscles are designed to work in pairs, flexing and extending in a kind of antagonistic partnership, with one muscle or set of muscles opposing another. For example, bend up your arm at the elbow. On the inside of the upper arm is the flexor, contracting as the arm bends upward. Its partner, on the outside of the upper arm, is the extensor, stretching or extending to complement the flexor's action. Put your fingers on them and you can feel the relationship.

To make this possible, muscle tissue has special qualities that enable it to change shape. It can become shorter and thicker (contractility); it can extend (extensility); and it can return to its original shape (elasticity). It also has an extremely important quality called tone.

"Tone" is a somewhat misunderstood term. Often it's used to describe a muscle's strength, or the way it looks or feels to the touch (a flabby muscle is said to have poor tone). Strength and appearance are related to tone, but in a technical sense tone refers to the property of muscle tissue which, when the muscle is healthy and in good working order, keeps it in a constant state of mild contraction. The tone of skeletal muscles contributes to their firmness, and maintaining a slight, continual pull on their attachments keeps the whole organism in a condition where it is ready to be responsive to the demands made on it.

Muscles have different degrees of tone, according to their purposes. Understandably, those with the highest degree are the so-called antigravity muscles along the neck and down the spine, which have the heavy work of helping us hold ourselves upright and maintain posture without a constant sense of fatigue. We've seen from our look at the spine that weakness in these muscles is not the only cause of back pain. But if they aren't equal to their task, they can provoke plenty of problems.

As we have said, it's only by improving the shape and condition of our muscles that we can affect the shape of our bodies. Exercise will improve elasticity and tone, and as the muscles respond it becomes increasingly possible for them to improve in three fundamental capacities that affect not only our looks but our overall fitness: muscular strength, endurance, and flexibility.

Muscular strength shouldn't conjure up a vision of the Incredible Hulk. In our context, it has nothing to do with exceptional strength or huge biceps. It is simply a term used for the amount of force that one of your muscles can produce in a single contraction. You don't need machines to measure your capacity. The ordinary tasks of everyday life are your gauge. You can't expect to be able to push a stalled car uphill, but you can expect to carry home your groceries, pick up a small child or a medium-sized suitcase, shove your way out of a crowded subway car, or kick open a jammed door—common demands that call for a reasonable degree of strength anybody ought to be able to exert when necessary. Apart from any special strength you might wish to develop to enjoy a particular sport, all your quota of muscle strength has to do is meet the reasonable needs of your life.

Exercise will develop the strength of your muscles; exercise with carefully calibrated weights (see page 102) will do it more quickly. It's not possible, with our quite unrigorous routines, that you'll develop any muscle so much that a difference in size will be visible. Firmness and responsiveness are what we're after. But even if you go on to more strenuous exercises, science has good news that will allay any fears you might have about ending up with a Charles Atlas physique. There are women who are interested in building up their bodies and are working at it, and as time goes by their muscles will respond and enlarge and gain the power they desire. But even the bodies of these women, the experts tell us, will probably never bulge in the way an overdeveloped male body can be made to bulge. Female glands apparently don't provide for that kind of enlargement; the male hormone testosterone seems to have a lot to do with it.

Your muscular endurance is simply the measure of the length of time over which you can repeat or sustain a particular muscular activity. You can talk about this in terms of how many leg lifts or pelvic tilts you can do, but what you're really concerned with is the practical operation of this endurance, how adequate it is in the reasonable course of your ordinary needs. For example, if you were a dedicated mountain climber and you slipped, you would have to be able to hang onto your rope until either you got your footing back or rescue arrived. Presumably you would have trained for years for this possibility; the muscular endurance called for is a good deal more than average. And in fact—exaggeration aside—if you are ambitious and go on to excel in some particular sport like swimming or tennis, you'll find it essential to work first on exercises that will develop not only your general endurance, but greater endurance in the muscles that will be especially involved.

However, standing up all day in a shop requires leg and back endurance. Office workers need endurance in their arms, necks, and backs if they want to make it to day's end without crumpling. If you have the muscular strength to push a lawnmower, but can only keep it up for five minutes at a time, your muscular endurance is less then it should be. Try the lawnmower again after you've done our exercises for a couple of months.

Flexibility is not precisely a property of the muscles. Technically, it's the degree of movement (called "range of motion") possible at the joints. Muscles are involved because the joint cannot move to its fullest unless its related muscles, tendons, and ligaments are all working together to their limits to support and extend to the joint's capacity.

Good flexibility makes all movement smoother, helps the body to absorb jolts, and reduces the vulnerability of body tissues to strains or tears. Slow, sustained stretching exercises improve flexibility. Do them for a few weeks, and then stretch up for something in a high kitchen cupboard which has always been a fraction out of reach. If you've been doing your homework well, you may be surprised.

What's so encouraging about muscles is that at almost any point in your life you can make up for past neglect and mistreatment if your demands are not unreasonable. Seventy-year-old ladies come into the YW's re-entry classes convinced they'll break in two if anyone so much as asks them to look to the right, much less to bend that way at the waist. Sometimes the instructor will even have them start their efforts sitting in a chair, and she'll proceed with great slowness and caution, guided partly by her experience and partly by the student's own "feel" for what she can and can't do. But however it starts and at whatever pace it proceeds, at the end of her course that woman is doing things with her body she never dreamed would be possible. She has a new, snappy (and younger) self-image, based not on fantasy but on the fact that she moves better, has more vitality, and functions better internally. She'll never be a threat to Chris Evert Lloyd, but for that she would have to have started sixty years earlier—and in any case that's not her aim. Like you, all she wants is to live her life at a better pace; like you, she is learning how much exercise can help her to do it.

Short of taking off a year for concentrated study, there's no way to learn all, or even a lot, about our muscular system. On the following pages is a capsulized view of the muscle areas that will be primarily involved in your exercises. Some idea of what this under-the-skin equipment looks like and how it works as you move is important to getting the most out of the time and effort you're planning to invest.

Neck, Shoulders, Back

Muscles in this area are primarily responsible for holding the neck and back erect, keeping the shoulders straight and properly aligned, and for some degree of arm movement. Misused, they lead to sagging shoulders and eventual humped back, double chin, and back problems.

Sternocleidomastoid muscles climb up the back of the neck to help hold the head erect and enable it to bend up and down and from side to side. When in good shape, they keep the neck slender and flexible and help achieve good posture. Proper exercise helps them combat the tension generated by the constant work of holding up the head, which weighs about twenty pounds.

The sacrospinalis muscle stretches up the length of the back, keeping the spinal column erect, strong, and flexible. It splits

VERTEBRAL COLUMN

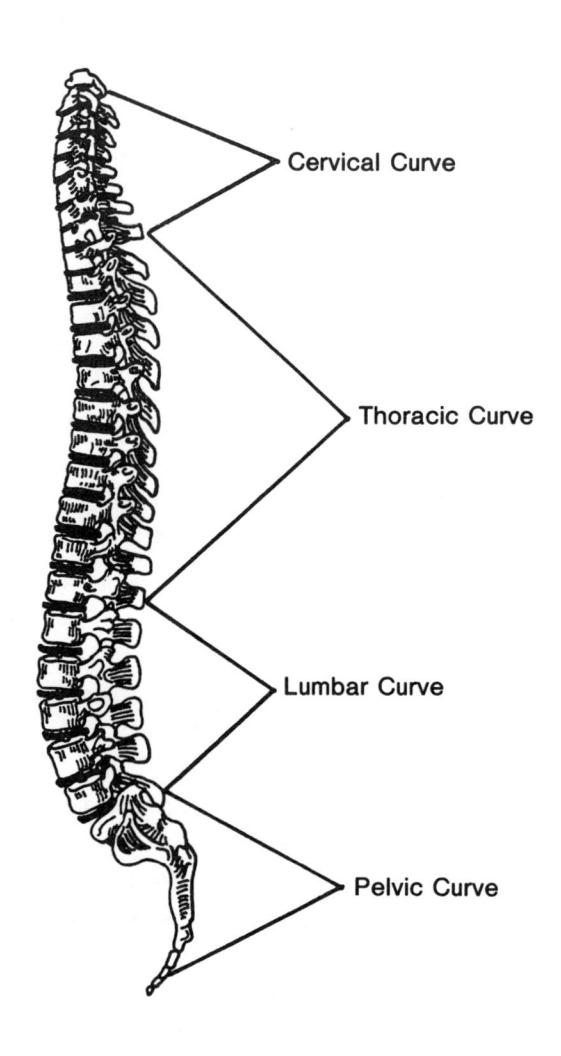

- Cervical Curve
- Thoracic Curve
- Lumbar Curve
- Pelvic Curve

into three sections as it climbs, with the sections attached to ribs and vertebrae at different points along the way. A strong, flexible back is dependent on these muscles; they are essential to keeping the vertebrae and spinal discs in proper alignment.

The latissimus dorsi and the trapezius are the broad muscles across the back, immediately under the skin, which assist in arm and shoulder movements. L. dorsi is the broadest and most powerful of the back muscles, extending in a flat triangle over the lower back. It aids in respiration by rasing the ribs; it joins with other abdominal muscles to pull the trunk upward; it operates to draw the arm downward and backward and also rotates it inward. Together with the abdominal muscles of the front, it contributes to a slender waistline.

The trapezius covers most of the upper back and neck. It raises the arms sideways and above shoulder level; it also lifts the head back and to either side.

Rhomboideus and levator, two upper back muscles that lie beneath the trapezius, are crucial to good posture. Both run from the spine to the edge of each shoulder blade (scapula). The two work together with the trapezius to raise the shoulder blades, draw them together, and flatten them. This in turn helps to draw the spine up, expand the chest, and flatten and straighten the upper back area.

Serratus anterior muscles lie horizontally along the ribs at either side of the body. They are positioned immediately beneath the skin and can be seen clearly when the arms are raised. Forward movement of the arms and shoulders brings these muscles into play.

Arms, Chest

What usually concerns women about the arm area is the flabby back of the upper arm. Put this down to the gone-to-seed muscles called triceps. These are three-headed muscles that extend the forearm, working in opposition to the biceps. Every exercise that benefits the biceps tends to benefit the triceps as well.

Biceps, found in the front of the upper arms as well as in the legs, are so named because they are two-headed. They are responsible for flexing the elbows and for a certain amount of movement in the shoulders and hands. These are the muscles that bodybuilders like to develop into mountainous knobs, an activity that strengthens the arms but can also defeat its purpose by overdeveloping a muscle so much that it interferes with the muscles around it. Unless you get into bodybuilding later on, this isn't relevant; what is relevant here is the knowledge that exercise will very quickly strengthen and firm the biceps in anybody's arms so that they look and work the way they should, consequently tightening up the triceps as well.

Deltoids are the muscles that cover the tip of each shoulder down over the upper arm, running across the shoulder joint. They are involved in all raising, lowering, backward, and forward movements of the arm. Loss of any portion of the deltoid interferes even with feeding and dressing.

Pectoralis, the breast muscle, covers the whole of the upper chest, extending over the upper ribs to the upper arm. Tightening the pectoralis raises the breast, an effect you can see at once in several of the exercises. A taut and elastic pectoralis is essential to a good bustline and posture. It is also important in arm movements, and to some extent defines the contours of shoulders and neck.

Abdominals

Most probably, if you could work on only one area of the body, this would be it. It's known variously as "nature's corset" or "nature's girdle" and with good reason, because when all its enormously complicated muscle groups are fit, they create a taut, nonbulging frontal outline and also do a lot of very serious undercover work for your spine (see page 36).

The principal abdominals are arranged in such a way that they form a three-layered shield over the front of the body from ribs to crotch. The most superficial (in the sense of being nearest to the surface) and the strongest are the external obliques. They are attached to the lower eight ribs and extend downward to terminating attachments in the pelvic bones, thus covering the whole front of the abdomen. Behind them are the internal obliques, whose fibers follow an opposite course, ascending from their origin in the pelvic area upward to their final attachment to the lower six ribs. Just beneath the internals are the transversus muscles, whose fibers are arranged horizontally and basically go from back to front. Situated forward in the abdomen is the rectus abdominis, which extends from the front of the pubic bone upward to the fifth, sixth, and seventh ribs. Its fibers are vertical, supporting the up-and-down direction of the external and internal obliques.

If you think of the abdominals as straps crossing and crisscrossing your abdomen, you'll see that they have to be toned not only up and down, but side to side, diagonally, and front to back, or back to front—if you get good enough at your exercises to work your muscles that deeply. As you can see, it's not just a matter of "holding your stomach in." But when they work properly, these muscles help to maintain a slender, youthful abdomen, keep the chest high, work hand-in-glove with the back muscles, and vitalize breathing, digestion and excretion. The exercises that accomplish this are a small price to pay for such results.

Pelvic Girdle (Hips, Thighs, Gluteals)

The pelvic girdle is actually the foundation for the spinal column. Through it, your weight is transmitted from your trunk to your legs, so its balance is vital. The muscles in this area control the alignment of the pelvis with the back, and, together with the thigh and gluteal muscles, affect the shape, size, and strength of hips, thighs, and buttocks. Among other functions, these muscles are responsible for our ability to lift our thighs and to rotate them inward and outward.

The inner thigh muscle, like that on the back of the upper arm, gets very little exercise ordinarily, unless our jobs call for a great deal of lifting, flexing, or squatting. For that reason these inner thigh and upper arm areas sag and grow flabby often before other parts of the body have begun to show signs of deterioration.

When you raise your leg, the muscle that you can feel on the front of the thigh is the rectus femoris, part of the quadriceps femoris, a four-headed muscle whose fibers unite at the lower portion of the thigh to form an exceptionally strong tendon. Opposing the rectus femoris at the back of the thigh is the biceps femoris. This is part of the group of extensors popularly called the hamstring muscles because the tendons that join them to the thigh bone are called the hamstrings. Hamstrings, both muscles and tendons, can cause a lot of trouble if allowed to stiffen, and their tone can be seriously damaged by poorly chosen footwear— generally very high heels worn for too long.

There are actually three sets of gluteal muscles (minimus, medius, and maximus) and, in addition to interfacing with the pelvic and thigh muscles, they contribute to firming your buttocks. Gluteus maximus is the largest of these muscles, but it takes all three working together to produce a neat, tight seat. We can give them more help than we realize, even without special exercises.

Now and then in the course of your day try consciously tightening and relaxing your buttocks. It's not a movement you can make just anywhere, anytime; you'll have to use your judgment. But it gives those normally mashed-down, underused muscles a little extra workout which, in conjunction with the exercises, can redesign your buttocks to a surprising and gratifying degree.

Lower Leg, Foot

Crucial in the basic action of walking—of flexing foot and ankle, moving legs, distributing weight—as well as in maintaining balance, are the muscles of the lower leg and foot.

At the front of the leg, the tibialis anterior pulls the balance of the body forward and is lengthened and relaxed as we point the foot. Flexing the foot, we activate this muscle.

The calf muscles, gastrocnemius and soleus, are among the most important in all forms of motion—running, jumping, walking—and are also continually used for balance by pulling the body weight toward the back. In a sense they are opposed by the peroneus muscle, which extends downward from the knee along the outside of the leg, finally to be anchored beneath the sole of the foot at the base of the big toe—the ball of the foot. This almost unknown muscle is therefore at the very base of our bodies. It helps to maintain the arch of the foot. Its support is vital in bearing the whole of our body weight. Weakness here means that tiny footbones can lose their relationship to one another, causing untold problems not only to the feet themselves, but transferring pressure and misalignment to areas much higher up, which are normally not associated with the feet at all.

Badly chosen shoes, or the continual wearing of high heels, may not only abuse but can actually damage the calf muscles. They are sometimes contracted to such a degree that abrupt exercise will tear them. But they are highly responsive to gentle, persistent stretching routines. "Gentle" and "slow-paced" are the watchwords.

Chapter 3
Doing It

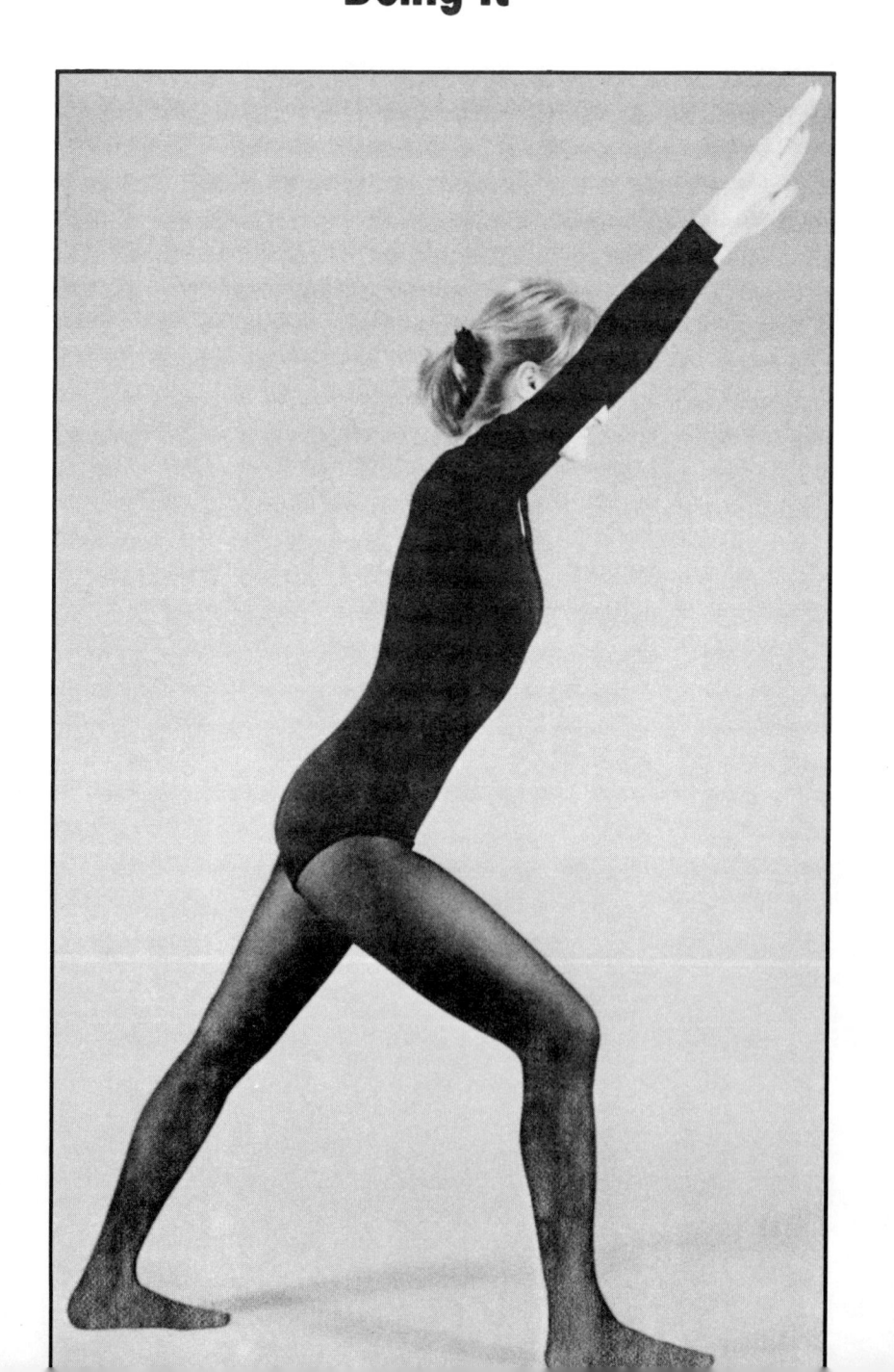

And now, to work. That's the right word. If we promised you nothing but fun, we'd be lying. We *can* promise, without reserve, that after a while you'll finish each session exhilarated by the activity.

But at the start, there's going to be a certain amount of teeth-gritting, plus some essential headwork you have to get through before you roll out your exercise mat. Bear in mind that, since you're contemplating a basic body-conditioning program—and that's the kind this book is all about—you're surely exercise poor. You're not a two-mile-a-day jogger. You've caught up with the fact that your body wants to move, *needs* to move, but there's a good chance it has forgotten how. You bulge and puff, you're frequently tired, sometimes depressed; in short, you're soggy in muscle and spirit.

However, you've picked up this book, which means that you've got the one thing going for you that's really what's needed: motivation. A desire to get back to working, feeling, and looking your best. You *make* a decision that you're tired of gasping for breath halfway up the stairs. You *make* a decision that you're fed up with looking the other way every time you catch your reflection in a store window. (This, and the three-way mirrors in dress departments, have brought more women close to suicide than broken love affairs.)

You've decided to embark on your own at-home conditioning program. Let's back off for a minute to point out that a class and an at-home program are not mutually exclusive. In fact, they're perfect partners. Generally, if you take a class, it's a once-a-week affair. Your instructor will confirm that exercising once a week, even for a full and strenuous hour, won't do what you're hoping for. It's not enough. Twice a week—well, better than once. Three times a week? Wonderful. But not many people can afford the time for three classes a week, not to mention the cost. So if you can take a class once a week and also support it with a daily workout on your own, you've achieved the perfect solution.

If no class is possible, this book can make all the difference—if you do your part. Take the trouble to learn carefully what to do. Do it faithfully, correctly, and honestly. These aren't just pep-talk words. They are guidelines without which you'll just be wasting your time. Observe them, and you'll get the results you're after. Furthermore, you'll be establishing a pattern that can serve you well for the rest of your life. That's because this YW program has been expertly conceived for that purpose by YW instructors who know from their years and variety of experience what women really will and will not do when it's up to them to do it on their own. There are no gimmicky twists, no faddish contortions, no elaborate routines that have to be restudied each time they're attempted. There's nothing for which you need blueprints or specifications. It has been well documented that tricky exercises are the first to go by the boards when there's no teacher standing over you to pull you along. Everything here is basic and can be done by you. It's tested, proven, performable by any average body.

This is the very nub of this YWCA body book. It is a program that has evolved out of years of leading thousands of women every week to a state of fitness.

It is based upon a series of basic routines with which you start and continue. Repetitions and pace mark the only difference between beginner and experienced practitioner.

It's one program for all bodies, with accent on the low risk factor. You will finish this 50-minute "YW" fitness course without danger of strain, soreness, or exhaustion from overdoing. In short, a total program. If you work, it works.

One Caution

Note above that we specify average body. This means average in shape, equipment, and condition. If you have a chronic health problem (blood pressure, heart strain, diabetes, susceptible knees or other joints, most particularly any back problem), you are probably already in regular contact with your doctor. As a matter of course, check with him or her as to the advisability of your embarking on this program. Even if you're in ordinary good health, if you haven't had a checkup within the last six or eight months, take the trouble to see your doctor, or at least talk to him or her. This commonsense precaution, incidentally, should be routine when you're contemplating any abrupt change in your physical habits—exercise, a new diet, an Outward Bound vacation, even a serious hiking trip, when normally you walk no more than from your front door to the nearest bus stop. You'll probably be told that this program will do you nothing but good, but nevertheless you should get this medical go-ahead before you charge forward.

What To Do Before You Do Anything Else

Commit yourself. Treat your decision to do these exercises as a genuine, personal obligation, as binding as one you would make if you went somewhere, signed up for a course, and put your money down. You don't have to be grim about it. But you want results, which won't come about unless your effort is wholehearted and consistent. Accept the fact that there's no way to wish yourself back into shape. Only the *doing* is going to pull in the abdomen, tighten the thighs, jog up the circulation: the regular, all-stops-out, faithful performance. The YW instructors are pretty harsh about this. They feel that if you're signing on with the dilettante notion of doing a few turns when the mood strikes, or if you suspect you can't count on yourself to do, on schedule and with full effort, what you undertake to do, then it's better for you not to get started at all. Now and then, one week off and one week on, won't do a thing for you except create big disappointment.

Framework Your Plan

If you sign up for a class, you know where and when you're expected to show up and how long it will take. Do the same on your own. Take a realistic look at your day and decide on a time slot that can always, or normally, be used for exercise. For most people, mornings before breakfast work best. If you're one of those who can't stand straight until you've had breakfast, you'll need to postpone activity until at least half an hour after eating—an hour is preferable; if you work, this is generally impractical. Early evening before dinner then might be the right time for you. Obviously, only you can figure out where your hour, or half hour, or fifteen minutes will best fit. Nor is it written in stone that the time can't be altered now and then to suit the needs of a particular day—but only when unavoidable.

Find a space. We're not nitpicking when we urge you to leave nothing to chance. Somewhere in your living space, whether it's a ten-by-ten studio or a five-bedroom condo, there's an area long, wide, and high enough for you to stretch out lying down or standing up, free enough to swing your arms, private enough to be comfortable. Find it and, if you live with others, stake it out as your special place for the time you've decided to exercise. If you live alone—well, you know the answer to that. Just go and do it.

How often? In fairness, we should report that not all instructors insist on an every day schedule. A minimum of three times a week satisfies some; most advise that to really keep in shape you should exercise at least on alternate days, which is a bit more than three times a week and of course includes weekends. Even the President's Council on Physical Fitness accepts "substantial engagement three times a week" as adequate for maintaining good tone and function. So, if an every day program seems too rigorous, you have license from some of the experts to lighten up the load.

However, why ask yourself to rethink the commitment every morning? "Is this my exercise day?" can too easily become,

"Oh, I'll do it tomorrow." Maybe you will, maybe you won't. It's much better not to give yourself the out, especially at the beginning. Just do it every day, until the habit is firmly entrenched—and this is what we're after—and it goes right along with brushing your teeth and putting on your clothes (or taking them off, depending on the time of day you've settled on). Soon you'll find that if you've had to skip a day, you miss it.

How long for each session? Face facts. If you know well enough that asking yourself for an hour a day is asking too much, scale it down. An honest half hour (read more below about honesty) will do plenty for you. And if you find on some mixed-up day that fifteen minutes is all you've got, don't write if off with "Never mind, I'll skip today and double up tomorrow." Your body doesn't work that way. Far better to do the fifteen minutes, maintaining your program regularly, and worry about tomorrow when it comes. Beginning on page 109 are our Emergency Shape-Up exercises, which are taken from this program and organized so that you can keep up your state of fitness in about fifteen minutes. There is almost no day during which you can't find fifteen minutes to do your exercises.

One supplementary word about the occasional Emergency Shape-Up. You might prefer to choose your own favorites to work out with. Making sure you do something is more important than making yourself do particular things. But keep in mind that experienced instructors suspect that your least-favorite routines are usually the ones your body needs most and is consequently most reluctant to undertake. So question yourself when you're selecting, just as your instructor would do if she were standing over you.

Equip yourself sensibly. Take care with this. You probably won't be foolish enough to plunge into your sit-ups in street clothing, but go a step further. Assemble a real set of work clothes. This can be anything loose, comfortable, nonconstricting, and neat: an old bathing suit, a pair of shorty pajamas, a halter top and shorts. Nothing to restrict a full stretch of arms, legs, or waist;

nothing tight around neck or waist. By far the best outfit is the one you'd wear to a class, available quite inexpensively in any lingerie or hosiery department: a proper leotard and a pair of dancer's tights. Don't substitute panty hose, which are usually too tight and toe-constricting; better to leave the legs bare. Treating yourself to a special outfit helps you take a serious approach to each session. If you can keep your work clothes handy in your practice space, you're even further ahead.

Unless your space is thickly carpeted, pay close attention to this recommendation. Get yourself an exercise mat. It doesn't have to be oversized, luxurious, or covered in designer fabric; any sports shop or department store offers basic and perfectly adequate mats, and again, they can be inexpensive. Never work on a bare floor, or one that's thinly covered. Not only can your knee and elbow joints become sore and abraded very quickly, but there's an unecessary chance of real injury if any part of you makes sudden contact with an unyielding surface. Maybe you work out next to your bed and can just slide the mat under it between sessions. Failing all else, try to leave the mat rolled up and handy to your space. Like all our other framework suggestions, it's a matter of getting all possible roadblocks out of the straight and narrow path between your resolution to do your exercises and your actual doing of them.

Now, the matter of weights. These have nothing to do with weight lifting, as in the Olympics. What we're talking about are two simple devices: broad braceletlike tubes of plastic filled with small metal pellets, which fasten around the ankles with Velcro tabs, and a pair of plain old-fashioned but lightweight dumbbells. The principle behind these weights is that they add to the weight of your own arms and legs. By asking the muscles to cope with this heavier-than-normal weight load as they contract and extend, these weights intensify the effects of the exercises performed with them.

You may use both ankle weights and dumbbells, but no rule says you must. You can work out with dumbbells alone or ankle weights alone, as well as both together. In all combinations, they're being used increasingly often these days in both men's and women's exercise classes because they seem to speed up many of the benefits one is working for: greater muscle strength and endurance, firmer contours, a more secure sense of being able to take care of oneself in a crisis.

Don't be concerned that you'll wake up one morning with baseball-sized biceps. Out of the selection available at your sporting-goods store, the only weights advisable for you to use are the lightest—two to two-and-a-half pounds for each dumbbell, the same for each ankle weight. This minimal additional load won't do a thing to your muscles except firm and strengthen them, probably at a faster rate than you'll achieve without them. In any case, female hormones make it almost impossible for a woman to come out of any exercise program with muscle-bound arms and legs, even if she's a serious weight lifter, which you're not—at least, not yet.

If you want to experiment with weights, be careful not to go over the poundage we suggest. Two and a half pounds in each hand or on each ankle is a total of five pounds of extra load, and that's absolutely all you should attempt at this stage. Also, don't rush ahead and use weights in all your exercises. You could put unwise strain on your back or neck by taking a wholesale approach. As you go through the exercises, you'll note that we've marked the ones that lend themselves best to working out with weights. Try those and see how it goes—but not until you have built up your stamina by several weeks of practice without weights.

The Guidelines Make the Difference

All right. You've sworn your oath. You've set up your schedule, you're wearing your leotard (which looks pretty good, considering, and think how much better it's going to look in a couple of weeks!), and there's your mat, ready.

Read through each routine from start to finish, much as you

would a recipe. You need to know what it involves, what it will require of you, and what it's aiming for overall. The instructions are broken down into steps that can't be misunderstood. After you've read them, do each one a few times. At the beginning, you will have to make a conscious effort to memorize them. Make it, and get the details right. They're important. Don't do any of these exercises casually. There's a reason for every movement. For example: In the first exercise you turn your palms forward before you raise your arms. That's so you'll end that movement with palms facing one another, involving different upper arm muscles than would be stretched if the palms faced out.

Do them honestly. *Honestly?* Surely an odd word in this context? Not for a minute. What it means here is: no faking. We can all fake far more cleverly than we like to admit; sometimes even the instructor (whose eyes, however sharp, can't be everywhere, every second, in a class with twelve, eighteen, twenty bodies to monitor) will be deceived by a stretched leg that looks as though it's fully extended but isn't, or a waist-bend that looks as though it's as far over as that particular body can go. Example: Stretch your arms up over your head. You can do it by raising the arms in a graceful but languid curve, elbows loose, wrists soft. Or you can genuinely stretch: feet planted for balance, spine pulling up out of the pelvic girdle, rib cage raised, shoulders down, straight arms pushing up toward the sky. In the first case, you're putting in practically zero effort, and the benefit from the exercise is zero. In the second, you're giving the whole body a fundamental stretch, tightening the waistline, opening the lungs, relieving tension. Your body knows the difference, and as you've already learned, what your body knows, it sooner or later tells.

So do each routine conscientiously. Do it full strength. Don't fool around with less than your best.

Ground Rules and Safety Nets

As we've said, these exercises ask nothing extraordinary of you. If you're in average good health, you can handle them without a worry. If your grandmother's in good health, *she* can handle them. That's the beauty of a program that's sensibly planned: You can go on with it for as many years as you care to. If you're feeling not quite up to par, scale down: do the short version, with fewer repeats. On the other hand, if you're looking ahead to a weekend of skiing or a tennis holiday, you can step up the pace at which you proceed and add repeats.

Though this program is as safe and simple as a whole department of specialists can make it, there are a few mild cautions that should be made part of your exercise pattern. They're mostly concerned with how and when it's wise *not* to exercise.

• Notice that "not quite up to par" doesn't mean flat on your back in bed. It doesn't have to be that bad. When you're nauseated, when your legs are weary, when your head is drumming like a set of bongos, forget Superwoman. Let your conscience guide you as to whether you're really incapable of exertion or are just copping out, and if it's the former, don't push it.

• Similarly, be mindful of the rule "Never work into pain." There used to be another phrase that went, "No pain, no gain," but that one has been discredited. Modern physical therapists caution that you must stop a movement at any moment when it begins to hurt. Leave it alone completely for a week, then try again gently. If it still hurts, either you're doing something wrong or that exercise is not for you. Wipe it out of your program.

• Your work space should be well ventilated, but be careful about drafts. A chill will stiffen a muscle faster than you might believe, and a stiff muscle is susceptible to pulling or tearing.

• For the same reason, *never* leap out of bed, or from any totally motionless condition, into any exercise routine. Your muscles, and your whole body, need to warm up gradually to the exertion. One student in pretty good general shape jumped up from a chair to answer the telephone and collapsed half-way with a torn soleus muscle in her calf. Considering this, we have not prescribed any exercises designated as warm-ups, because our first few routines require such moderate activity that they serve the purpose. Nevertheless, we have assumed that before you get to your exercises you will have been walking around a bit, bending to pick up your shoes, setting a table, reaching up for a can of coffee. If this assumption doesn't fit the facts, you'll have to give warming up a bit of thought. Walk around the room, or the whole house if you've got one; go up and down the stairs; bend down and pick up those papers someone left lying on the floor. You don't have to paint the ceiling or climb Mt. Everest, just make sure you don't jerk your body from total repose into sudden exertion.

• After the last exercise, you're cautioned not to collapse in a heap, but rather to bring the body's activity to a gradual stop. This is because cooling down is as essential as warming up. During activity, the heart has been forcefully pumping blood into the muscles and respiration has increased. If the activity stops abruptly, there is no mechanism that can return the blood quickly to the heart, and it begins to pool in the muscles and veins; there is also a danger of faintness or light-headedness because oxygen-bearing blood is not returning quickly enough to the brain. When you bring your activity down gradually, the muscles have time to relax and expedite the return of blood to the heart and brain.

Also, after strenuous activity, a body waste called lactic acid forms in the muscles. Oxygen is needed to reduce this acid accumulation. A proper cool-down period helps to disperse the waste and thus minimizes any soreness and discomfort.

• Whatever exercise you're doing, be mindful of the lumbar area of your back—the five lumbar vertebrae and attendant muscles that make up the "small" of the back. This is important to remember *whatever* you're doing, not just when exercising. Its slight natural inward curve should never be permitted to intensify This leads to pelvic and leg pressures and inevitably causes an exaggerated forward droop of the abdomen; those muscles then become even weaker and more out of control. Many of the exercises, both standing and lying, will strengthen this area if done properly and were designed for that, but if you're careless about the constant admonition to "roll down" and "roll up" you can possibly put enough strain on this fairly weak area so that you hurt yourself. So be warned and be vigilant.

• Finally, not a caution but a cheerful bit of advice. Music. Remember that early days' "piano accompaniment"? You can work to various kinds of music. Choose something light and pleasing—rhythm-and-blues isn't for everyone. Most important, make it something with a sustained and insistent beat that will carry you along. You can work without music, but it's not as much fun, and you'll find that the momentum carries you along and keeps you from tiring quite as soon as you might otherwise.

You'll notice that the exercises begin with one for posture. Good posture—carrying your skeleton in the proper alignment to support your body—is not usually described as an exercise. But in this series it's of such fundamental importance that it's treated as one. In most of what follows you're constantly reminded to stand straight, stand tall, check your body alignment. But for the average harried, hurried, slouched, tensed-up body, doing this correctly involves so many adjustments that it really does become an exercise. The value of everything that follows depends on how diligently you work to get this right and keep it that way throughout to the best of your ability—which will increase amazingly as time (and practice) goes by.

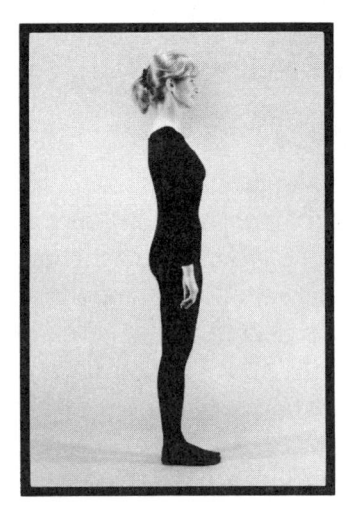

1 Posture

NO!

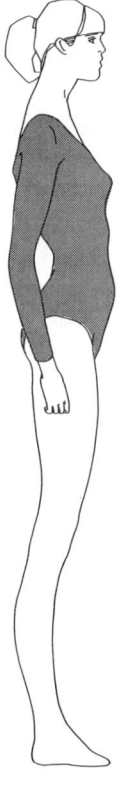

1 Balance the weight a bit forward, toward the balls of the feet. Don't lock the knees or bend them; they should be slightly relaxed.

2 Curl your tailbone under the buttocks. This brings the pelvic girdle a fraction down in back, up in front, which makes it easier to concentrate on the next step: pulling in the abdomen and pulling up the rib cage.

3 As you pull up, you run into trouble. The small of your back wants to curve forward. Don't let it. The key is to pull back and up at the waist, imagining as hard as you can that the front is going to come in so far it will touch the back. It will never happen, but that's what you visualize. Your buttocks will contract even further, and if you're watching in a mirror you'll get a flash of what your body could look like if you'd been doing the right things all along. Never mind. You're doing them now.

4 Keep pulling up hard. Feel the spine straighten. Actually think about pulling each vertebra up and away from the one below. Keep pulling up as the stretch climbs the back of your neck.

YES!

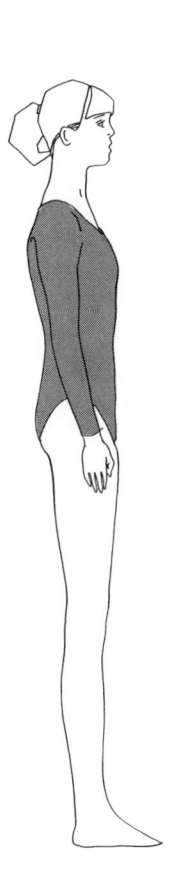

5 Don't let the shoulders rise. Keep them level and down. And don't squeeze them back; you're not after the chest-out stance of a West Point cadet on parade.

6 With ears over shoulders, continue the stretch to make your head come up, much as though a string at the back of it were pulling your head toward the ceiling. Keep the chin level.

7 If you're getting it right, you've taken up to two inches off your waist measurement and possibly gone up an inch in height, simply by standing the way you were meant to stand. You've also eliminated the sagging shoulders that give you that defeated look and made a good start in your war against the dreaded dowager's hump, that unsightly thickening that builds up at the back of the neck between the shoulder blades on a base of stretched muscle. For all these reasons, good posture is an exercise in itself.

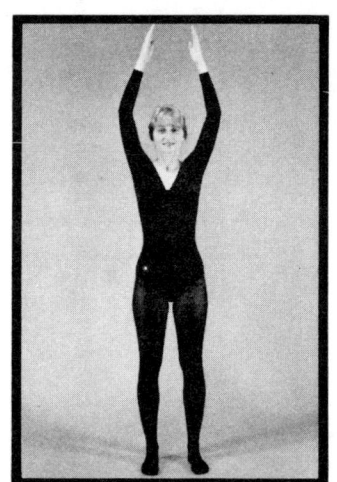

2 Structured Breathing (a)

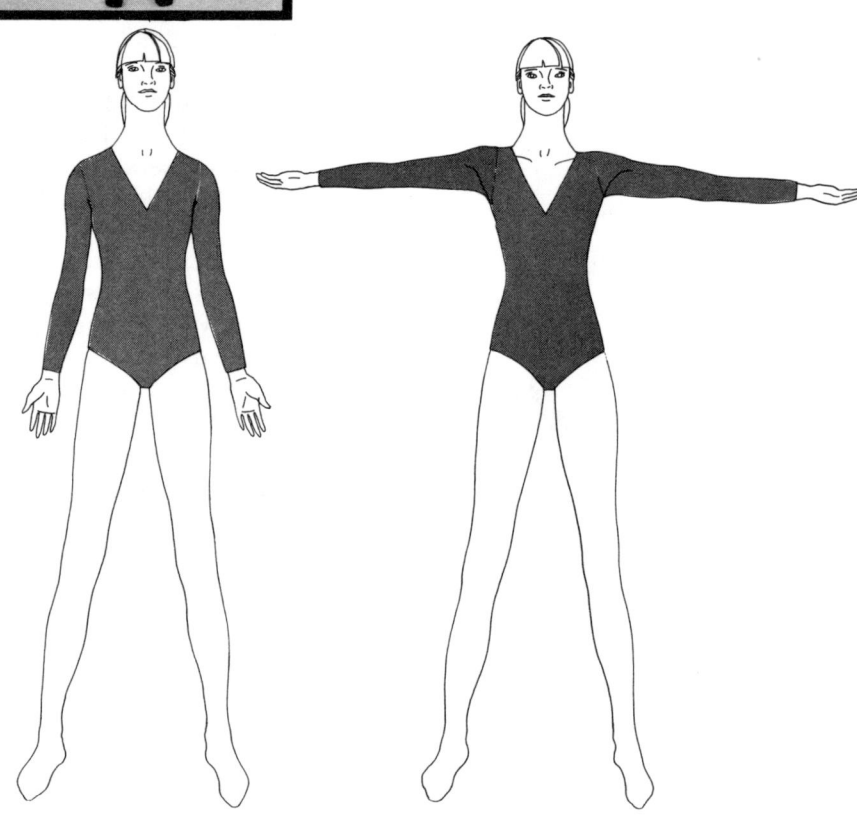

1 Stand with feet comfortably apart, knees loose but not bent, arms at sides. Turn palms forward. While inhaling to a slow count of 6, sweep arms out sideways and up over head so that palms face one another.

56

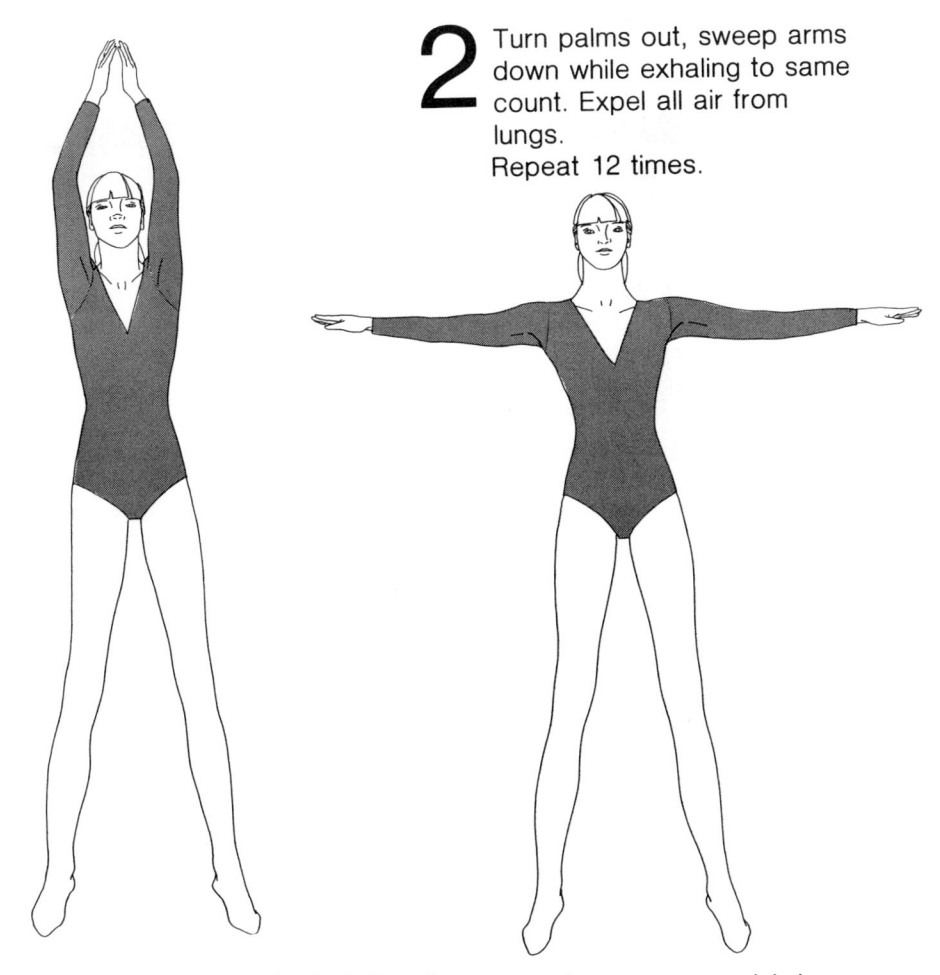

2 Turn palms out, sweep arms down while exhaling to same count. Expel all air from lungs.
Repeat 12 times.

As you become adept at the above exercise, you may wish to vary it with the following In that case, do only 6 repeats of Structured Breathing (b)

Structured Breathing (b)

1
2 Perform steps 1 and 2 as in Structured Breathing (a). Contract the abdominal muscles hard to push out the last bits of air. Hold the contraction for count of 3, and relax.
Repeat 6 times.

- **Maintain posture; make sure body does not bend on the exhalation.**
- **Keep count rhythmic and even.**

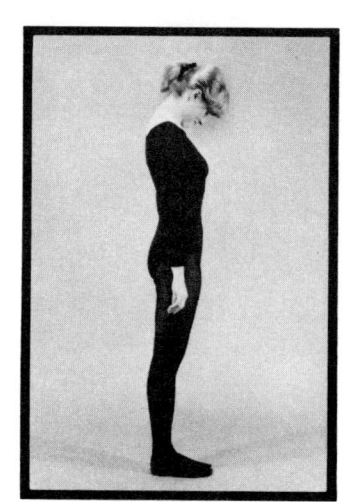

3 Chin Pendulum

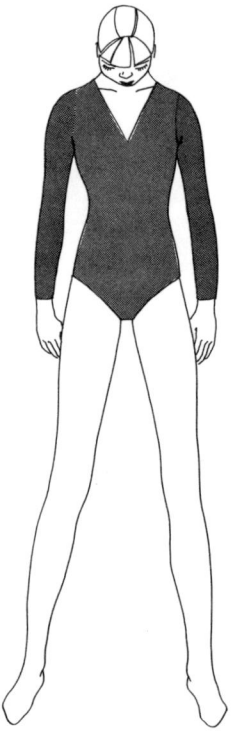

1 Drop chin toward chest, stretching back of neck. Keep shoulders down and back; do not bend body.

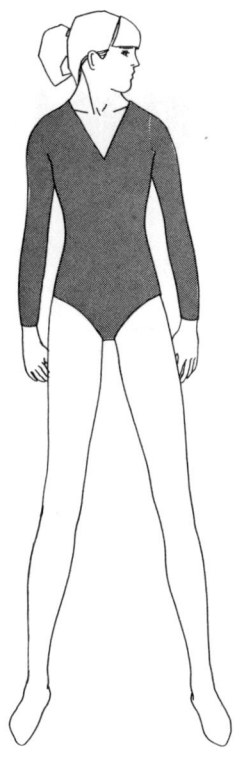

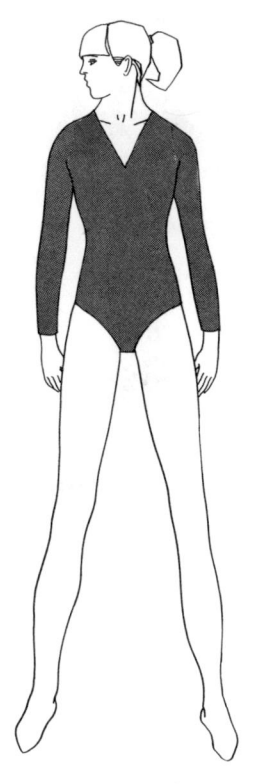

2 Keeping chin close to neck, move it slowly up toward left shoulder. Moving slowly and smoothly, bring it back down and up toward right shoulder Repeat 4 times to each side.

- **Don't push; though the back of the neck is stretched, the neck muscles should be relaxed so that the whole movement is relaxed and smooth.**
- **Don't force the chin any farther than is comfortable. If you can look out over the shoulder you're getting enough out of this exercise.**

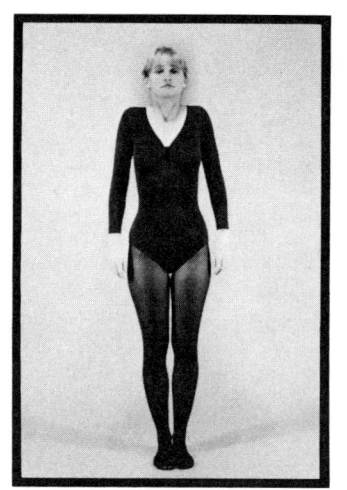

4 Shoulder Rolls

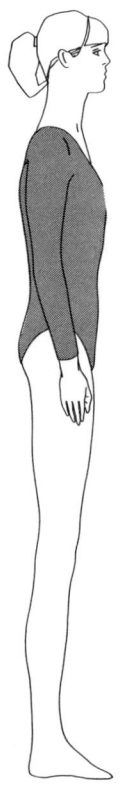

1 Stand relaxed, arms at sides. Keep neck tall.

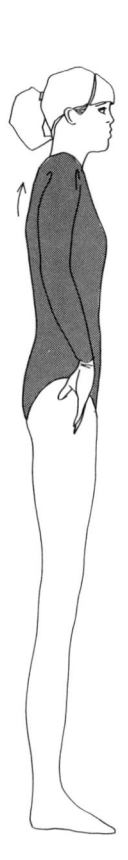

2 Bring shoulders up toward ears. Inhale on this motion.

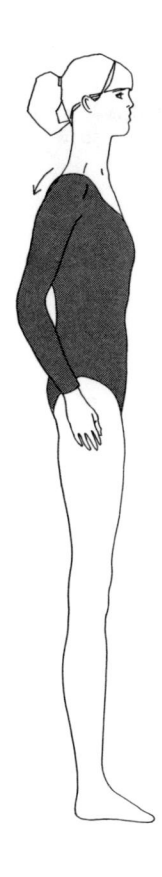

3 Roll shoulders back and down, exhaling as movement ends.
Repeat 8 times to slow count.

- **Don't bend body forward or allow head to drop forward.**
- **Only the shoulders are really in motion; however, since the arms are relaxed at sides, they will move slightly as the shoulders roll.**

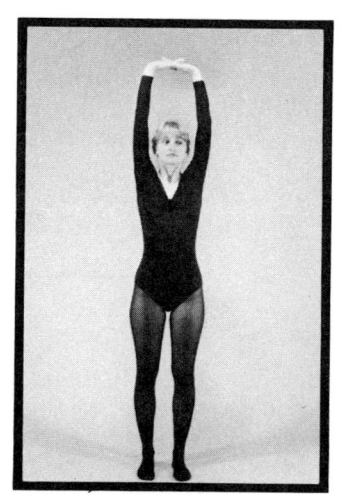

5 Arm Stretch

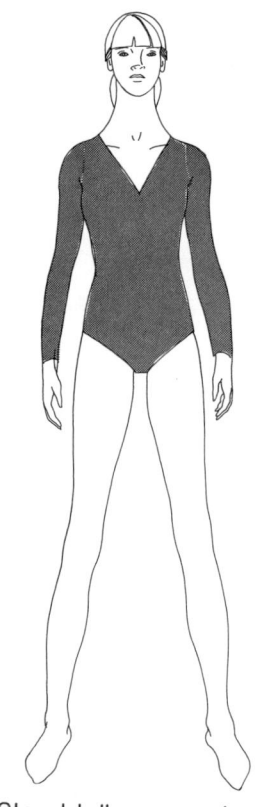

1 Stand tall, arms relaxed at sides, feet comfortably apart.

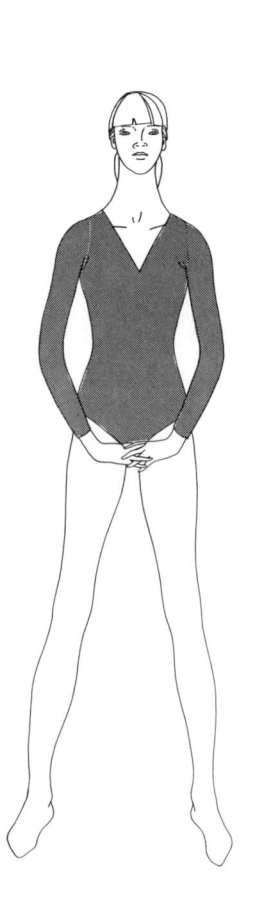

2 Bring hands together, intertwining fingers. Turn palms downward.

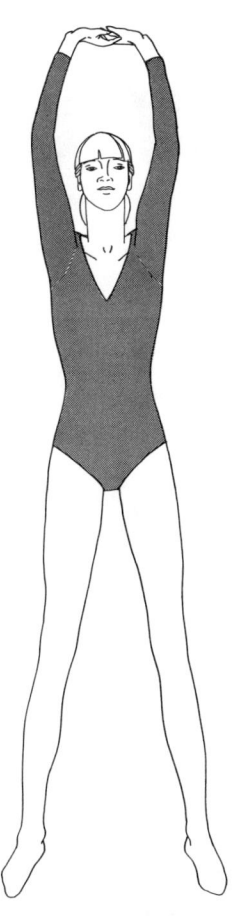

3 Inhale and swing clasped hands up overhead. Hold for count of 4. Keep elbows straight but not locked. Palms will be facing ceiling.

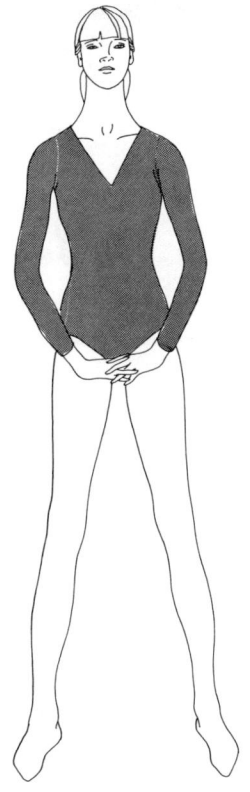

4 Face palms downward, fingers still intertwined. Bring arms back down as in illustration 2, exhaling on this movement.

5 Separate hands, return arms easily to sides.
Repeat 4 times.

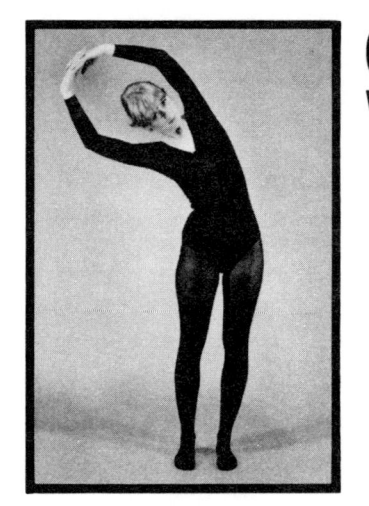

6 Waist Stretch

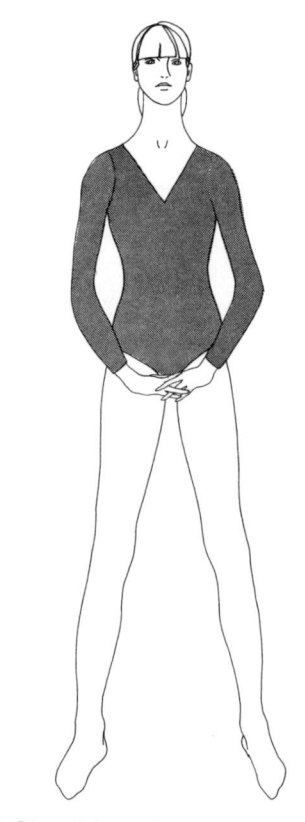

1 Stand tall. Clasp hands, palms downward.

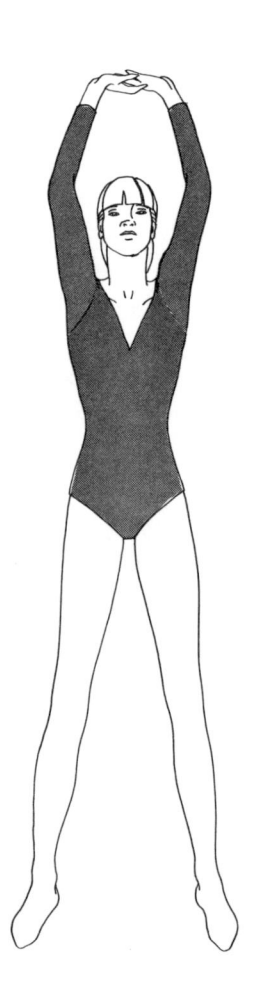

2 Swing arms up overhead.

3 Breathing normally, bend from the waist to the right as far as is comfortable, allowing clasped hands to lead the movement.

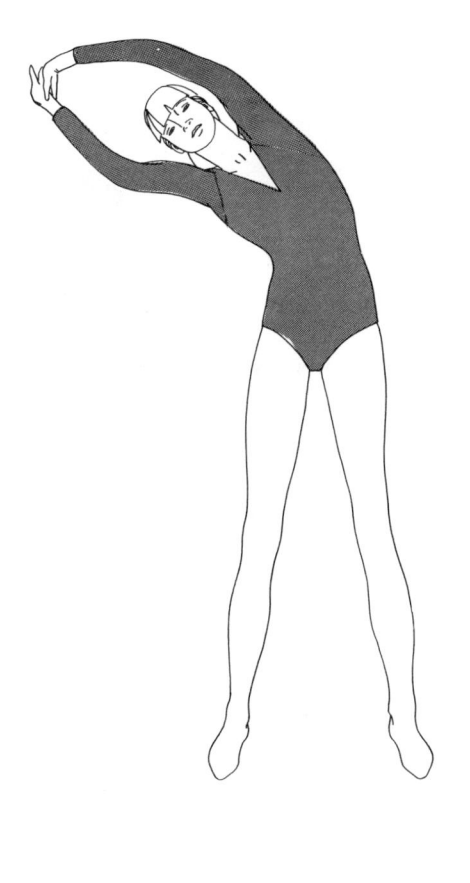

- **Feel the stretch in your waist, but don't force it beyond what is comfortable. As you practice this, your waist will become more flexible and you will bend further without forcing.**
- **Only the upper body moves; don't allow your hips to move out of alignment, or your knees to bend.**

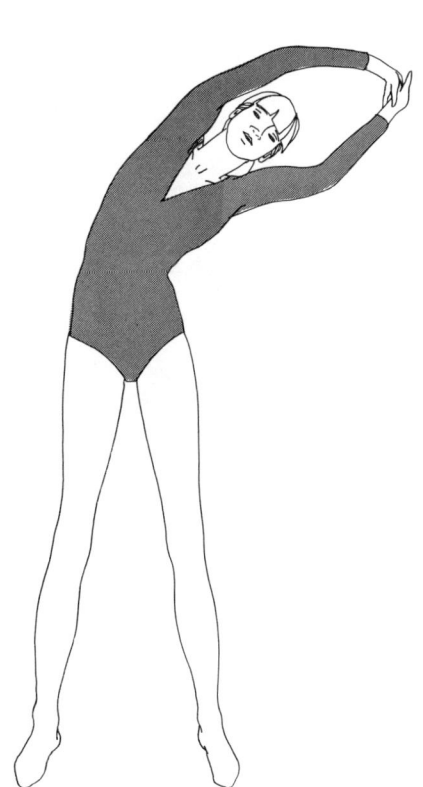

4 Straighten and repeat, bending to the left.
Repeat 4 times to each side.

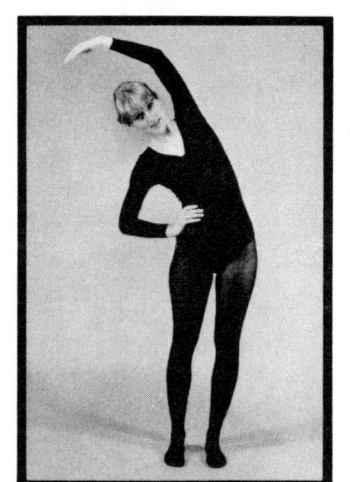

7 Waist Trim
●━●

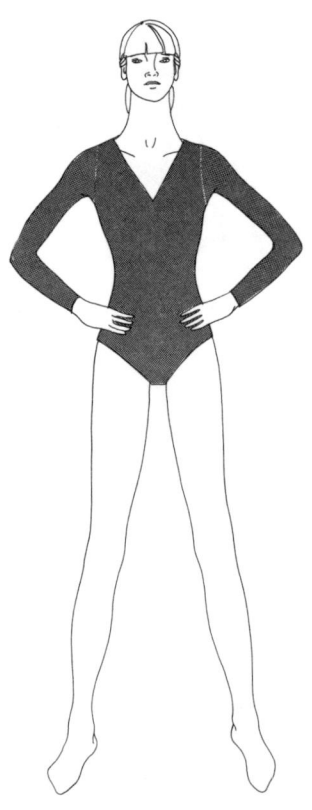

1 Stand tall, buttocks tucked under, abdomen pulled in. Place hands on hips, feet comfortably apart.

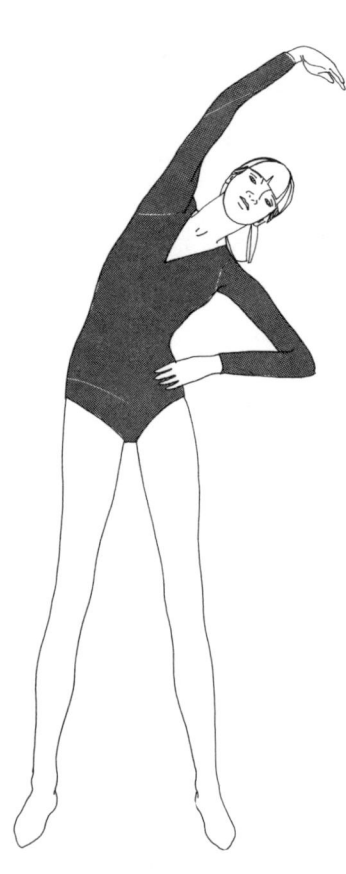

2 Swing right arm up past ear, curving it slightly. At the same time, bend from the waist to the left.

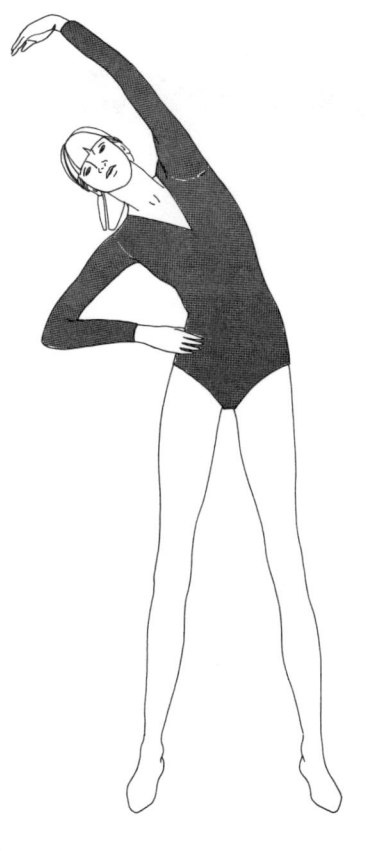

- **Breathe normally throughout this exercise.**
- **Maintain good body alignment throughout. Keep abdomen in, buttocks under.**
- **Don't allow the bend to bring the upper body forward. The arm goes up and over, and the upper body follows this line.**

3 Reach with the right arm toward the opposite wall, keeping the abdomen pulled in and feeling a good stretch along the right side down to the waist.

4 Return to level position, hands on hips.

5 Repeat, swinging left arm over to right side. Repeat, alternating arms, 8 times to each side.

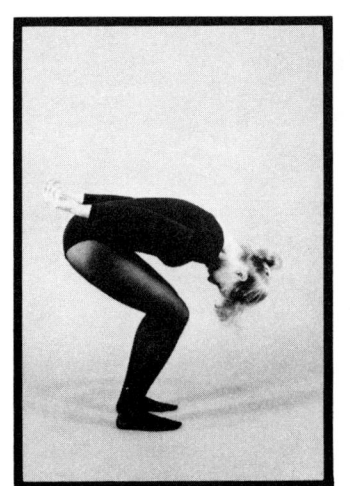

8 Body Swing

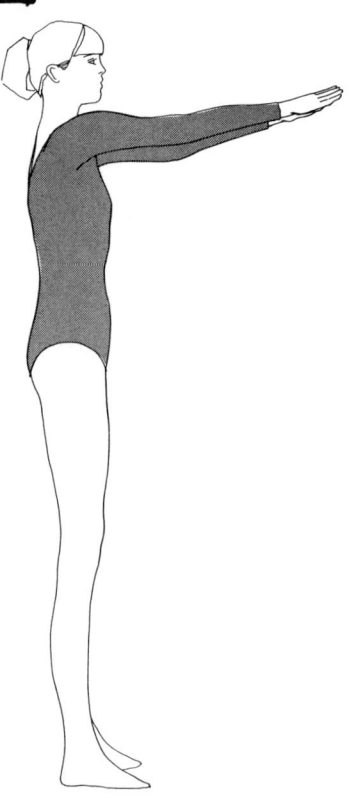

1 Stand relaxed, feet far enough apart for good balance, arms loose at sides. Swing arms forcefully forward to about shoulder level.

2 Simultaneously bend knees, drop head and upper body forward slightly, and swing arms forcefully downward, allowing the momentum of the swing to carry them well up in back. The body rocks slightly upward from the knees as the arms go back, but remains semicrouched.

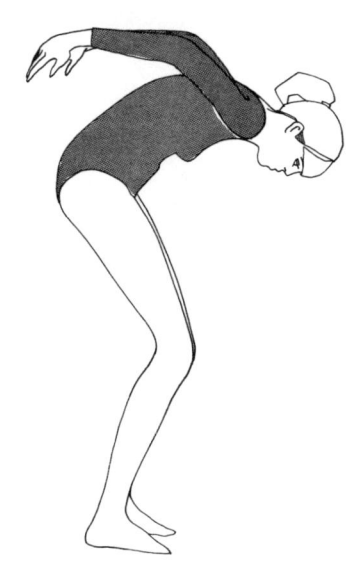

3 Swing arms forward and straighten body to standing position.
Repeat at least 6 times.

- This is a loose, continuous movement involving the whole body. Swing rhythmically.
- Keep the knees bent and springy so that they can follow the down-and-up movement of the arms, adding to the momentum.
- Think of a playground swing; that's the motion you're imitating.

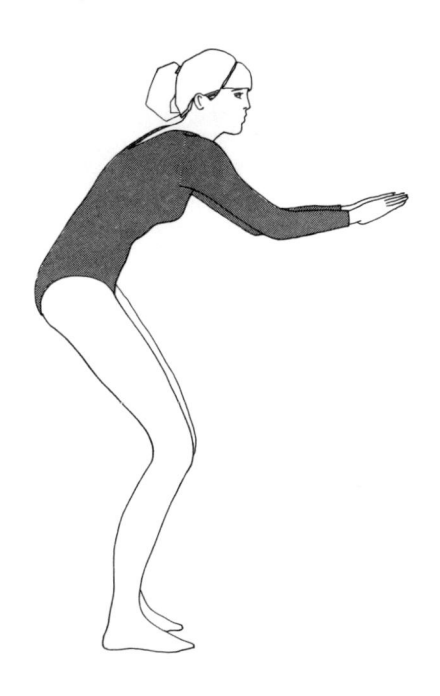

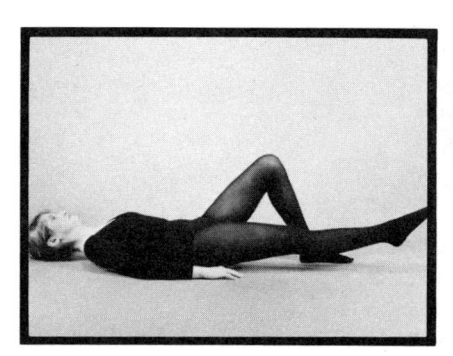

9 Leg Stretch

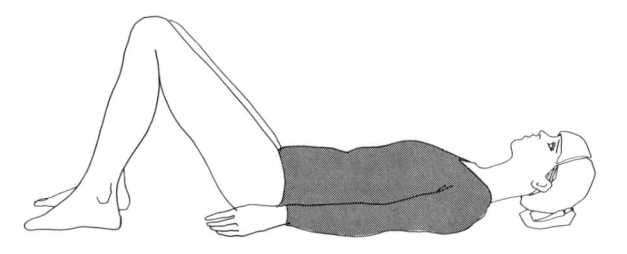

1 Lie flat on back, knees bent up, feet flat on mat at comfortable distance from hips and about hip-width apart. Press small of back down into mat; there should be no space between the small of your back and the mat.

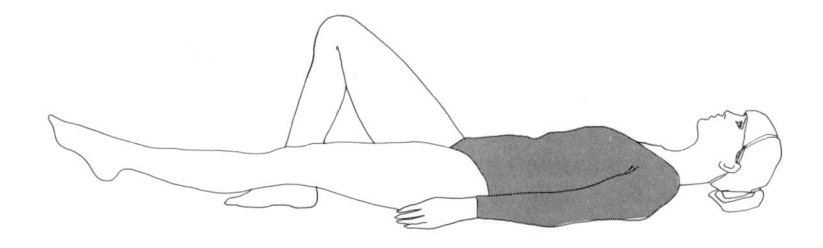

2 Straighten left leg out, holding it about 2 inches above mat.

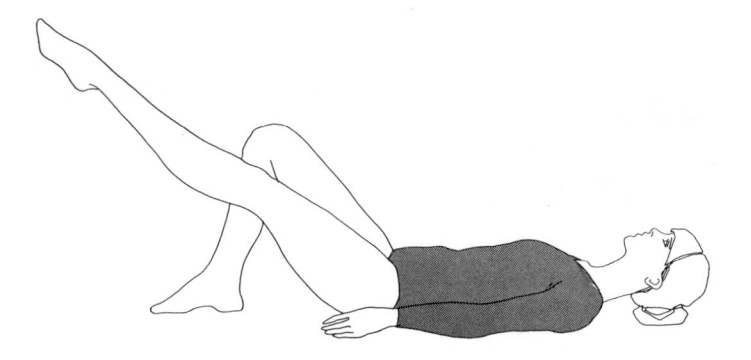

3 Lift left leg straight up to comfortable height, then lower to position 2. Inhale on upward movement, exhale on down, to a measured count of your own choosing.

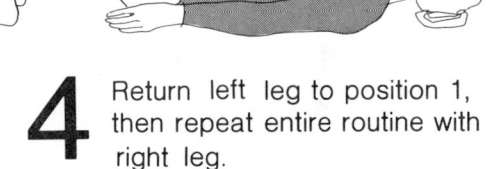

4 Return left leg to position 1, then repeat entire routine with right leg.

Do the above routine twice with each leg to start. After a few days, add 2 more lifts with each leg; then try to build up to 2 lifts more each day, until you are doing 8 lifts with each leg. Stay with this for a couple of weeks, then add a few more. You're working toward an optimum 16 lifts per leg, but there's no law about the number. Don't force yourself beyond what you can do comfortably.

• **Maintain straight body alignment throughout; also, keep the small of the back flat against the mat. This position is crucial in all flat-on-the-floor exercises; otherwise there is too much strain.**

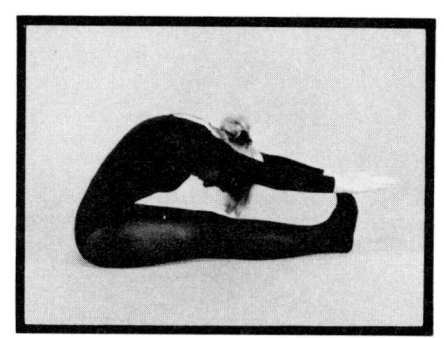

10 Spine Stretch

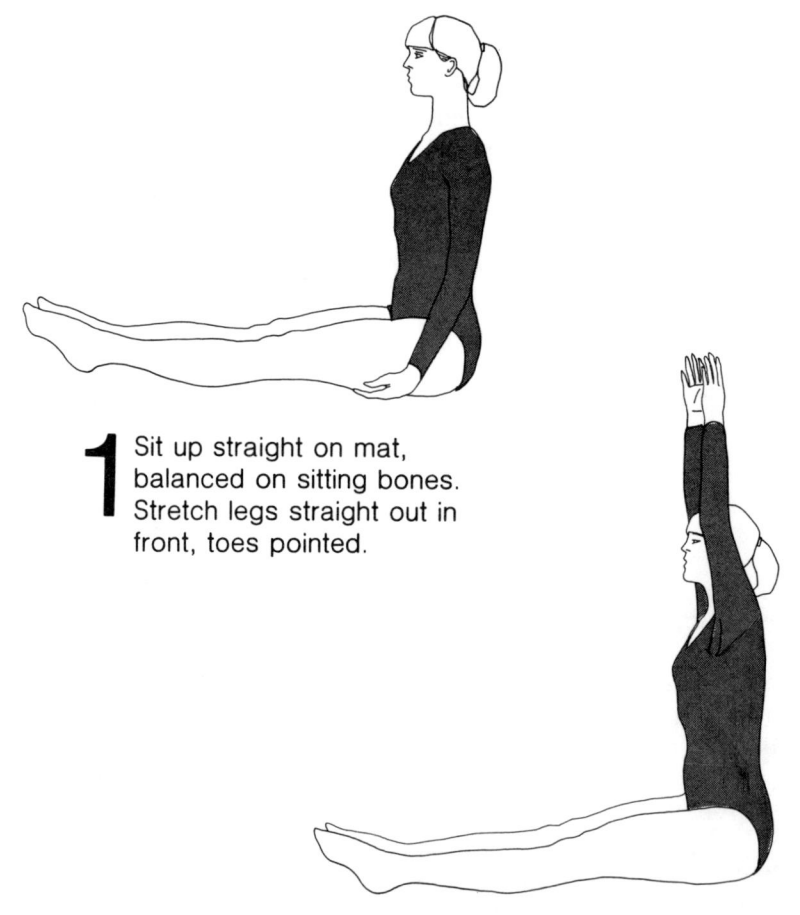

1 Sit up straight on mat, balanced on sitting bones. Stretch legs straight out in front, toes pointed.

2 Stretch arms up over head, reaching hard to lift rib cage. Keeping ears over shoulders, stretch neck up hard. Inhale on this movement, but make it a normal breath, not a deep inhalation.

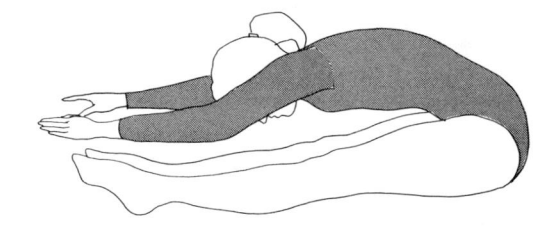

3 Drop chin toward chest to stretch the back of your neck. Simultaneously lower arms to shoulder level and bend body forward, arms reaching out over legs as far as possible. Exhale on this movement.

4 Return to position 1.
Repeat 8 times with toes pointed, then 8 times with feet flexed.

- **Don't try to reach your toes unless you can do it without strain. More flexibility will come in time. Eventually you will reach your toes, but this exercise does its work whether you reach your toes or not.**
- **Keep the knees and the arms straight throughout.**
- **After a few days, try to hold the last reach for a slow count of 6. This increases the value of the stretch.**

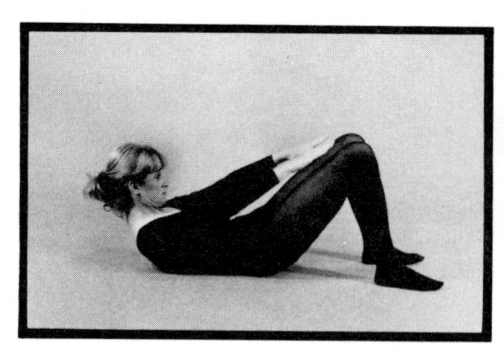

11 Modified Roll-up

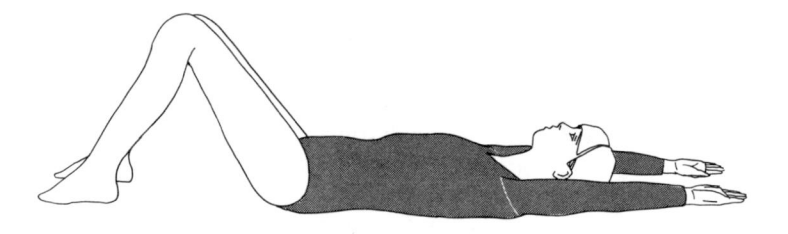

1 Lie flat on mat, knees bent up, feet flat on floor a comfortable distance from hips and about hip-width apart. Stretch arms back along mat.

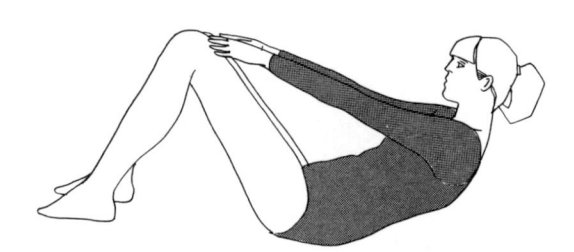

2 Reach arms up and over toward knees; simultaneously raise head and shoulders, but only as far as possible without strain.

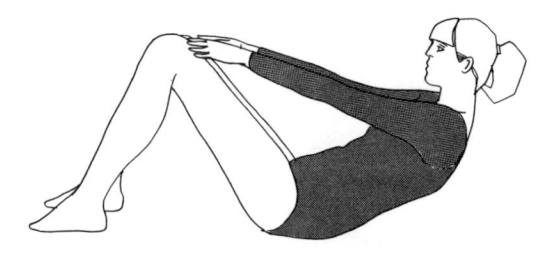

3 Roll down, feeling each vertebra in turn as it touches the mat.
Repeat 4 times at start; aim toward 8 as capacity increases.

- **Keep the small of the back against the mat.**
- **Use the muscles of the abdomen and diaphragm to help pull you up.**
- **Note that a full sit-up is not the object of this exercise. Pull yourself up only as far as possible without strain and without shifting position.**

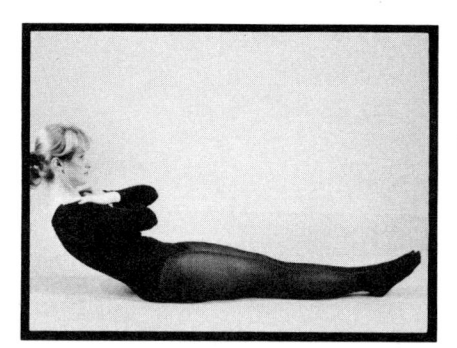

12
Sit-Up (a)

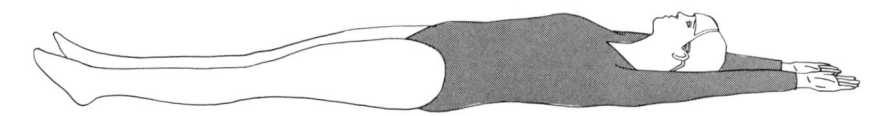

1 Lie flat on mat, arms stretched up overhead, small of back pressed down into mat, knees straight.

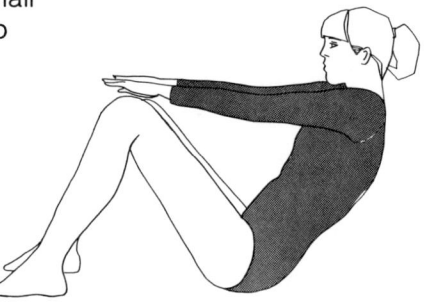

2 Swing arms up and forward, simultaneously raising body to sitting position. The momentum of the arms will get you up, but try also to employ the abdominal muscles, since that's the area you're trying to work with this exercise.

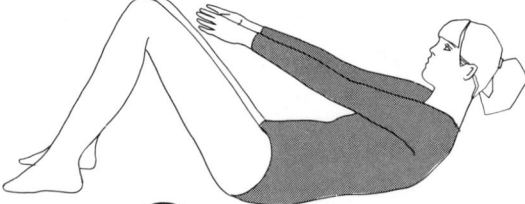

3 Roll down back to position 1.

Repeat 2 times at start. When you can do that without shifting or struggling, add 2 more each day until you are up to 8.

Sit-Up (b)

When you can comfortably do 8 of Sit-Up (a) start from a lying-down position with the arms resting alongside the body. Raise yourself to sitting position without using arms in any way. The abdominal muscles will have to do it all.
Repeat 2 times at start; then try as in the previous exercise to achieve 8 times.

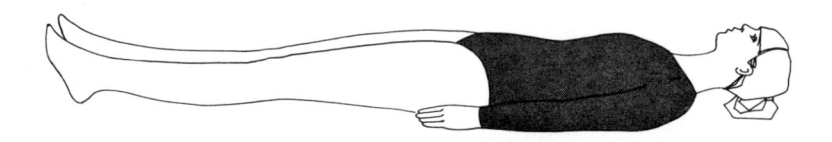

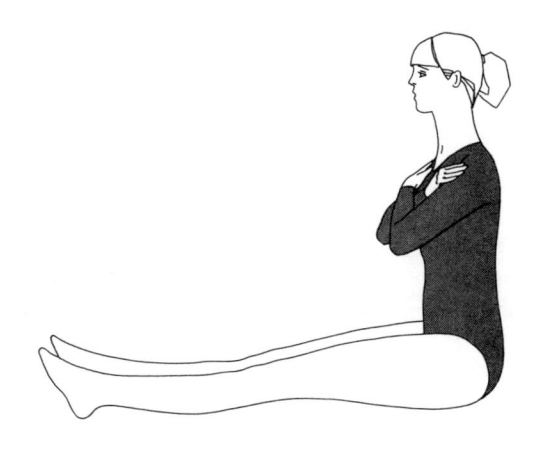

Sit-Up (c)

When Sit-Ups (a) and (b) have become child's play, start from a lying-down position with arms crossed over chest and raise yourself to sitting position.
Repeat 2 times at start, and advance to 8. When you can do this relatively easily, forget about (a) and (b) and do all sit-ups with the crossed-arms technique.

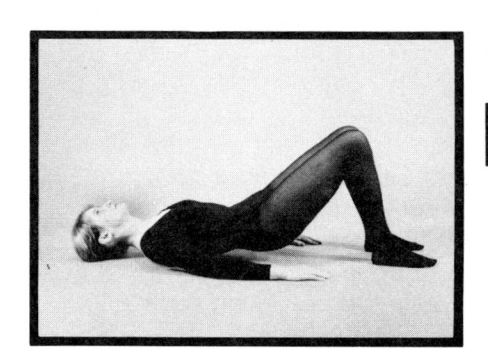

13 Pelvic Tilt

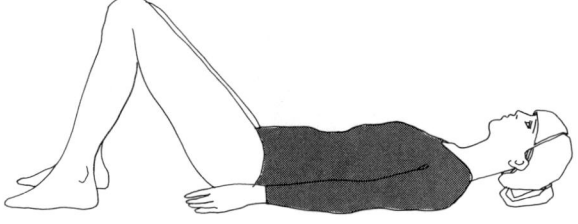

1 Lie flat on mat, arms at sides. Bend knees up, place feet flat on mat, parallel, about shoulder-width apart.

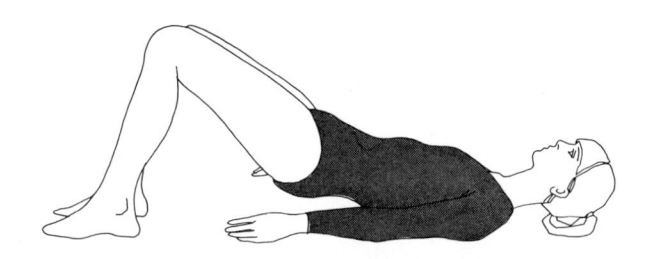

2 Contract buttocks. Curl tailbone under. This will raise hips slightly. Continue raising hips as far up as comfortable, while shoulders remain on mat. Keep spine straight. Hold position for a few counts.

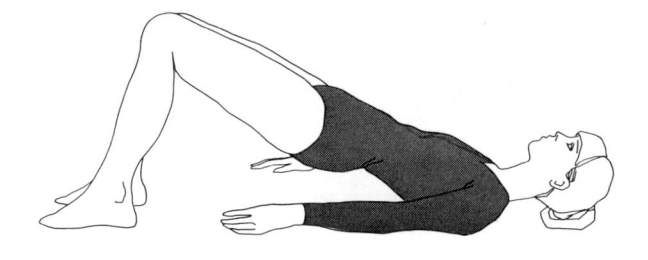

3 Be aware of cervical vertebrae pressing against mat. Then bring hips back down to mat by rolling spine down section by section, feeling pressure of each vertebra in turn against mat. Be sure small of back rolls down before hips touch mat.

4 Take a few normal breaths before repeating.
Repeat 2 times to start, adding lifts up to 8 as capacity increases.

- **Both lift and roll-down should be done slowly.**
- **Concentrate on the vertebra-by-vertebra roll-down coming down; it is crucial to this exercise.**
- **Breathe normally throughout.**
- **If you feel strain in the muscles at the back of the thighs, your heels are in too close to the body for your present capacity. Move them farther forward.**

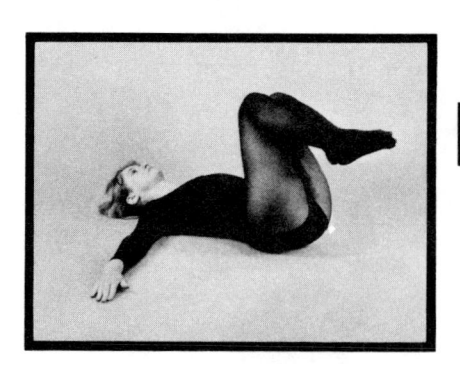

14 Hip Roll

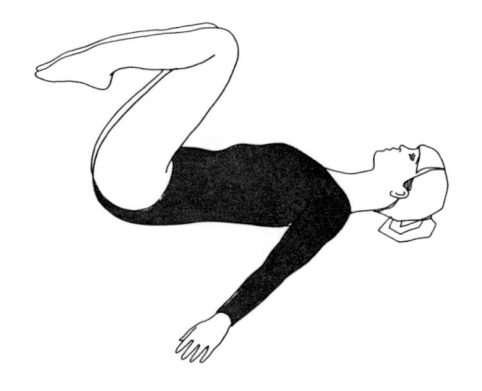

1 Lie flat on mat, body aligned, small of back flat, shoulders down, arms out sideways, palms down. Bring knees up to chest, or as far up as they will come without disrupting body alignment.

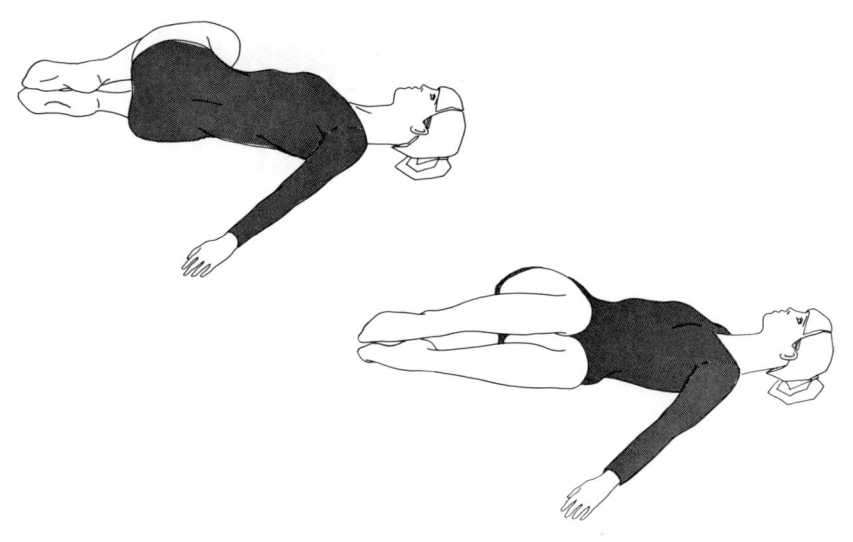

2 Keeping knees together, roll them to the right, then to the left, trying on each roll to touch the bottom knee to the mat. The hips will roll as the knees swing over, but keep the shoulders down and the spine straight.
Repeat 8 times to each side.

- **Breathe normally throughout.**
- **Concentrate on keeping the knees together, the shoulders down, and the small of the back flat against the mat. This means the abdomen will also be pulled in.**
- **You're aiming toward getting the bottom knee down on each roll, but don't force it. It's more important to keep your knees together and keep your spine in straight alignment. More flexibility will come in time.**

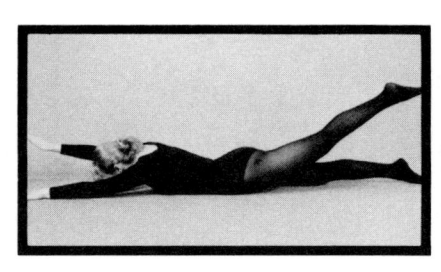

15 Alternating Stretch

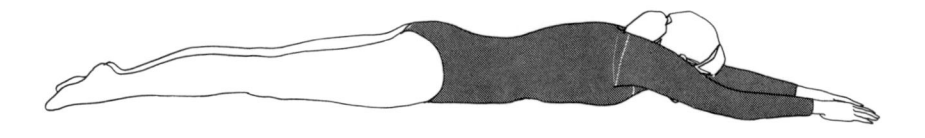

1 Lie flat on stomach, chin on mat, arms extended forward, legs straight back, toes pointed but relaxed.

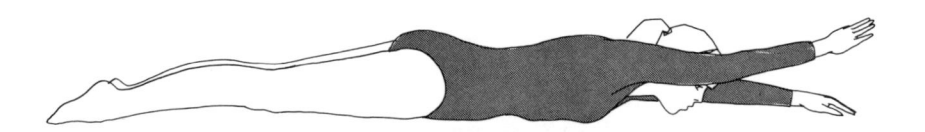

2 Keeping chin on mat, raise right arm as high as it will comfortably go. Return it to mat, repeat with left arm.

3 Alternating the arms, do 4 lifts with each arm. Then return to position 1.

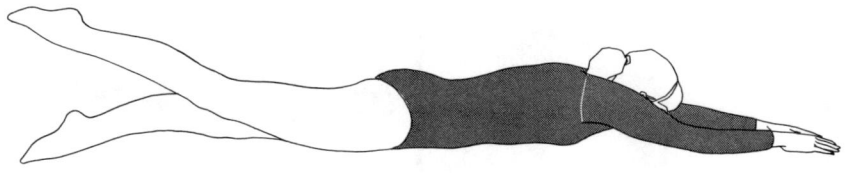

4 Keeping hipbone on mat, raise right leg from hip to comfortable height. Be sure to keep knee straight. Return it to mat, repeat with left leg.

5 Alternating legs, do 4 lifts with each leg. Return to position 1.

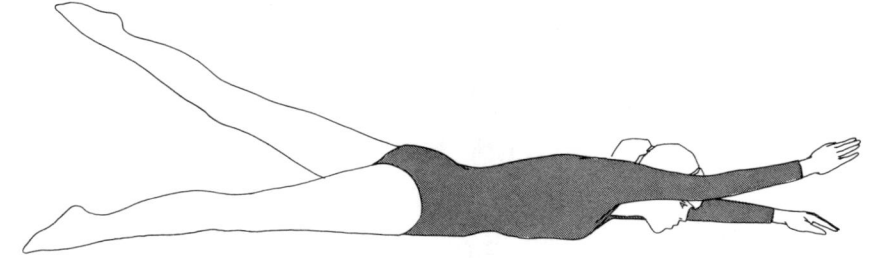

6 Simultaneously, lift right arm and left leg and return them to mat. Keep chin and hipbone against mat.

7 Repeat with left arm, right leg. Return to mat. Repeat each arm-leg combination 4 times.

- **Don't strain to lift any higher than is comfortable.**
- **Inhale with each lift; exhale as you come down.**
- **Don't allow the body to roll over; it will have a tendency to do so if the hipbones do not remain on the mat.**

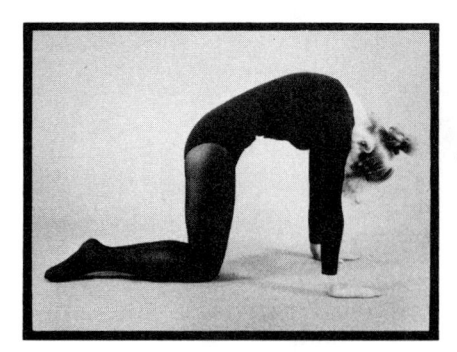

16 Angry Cat

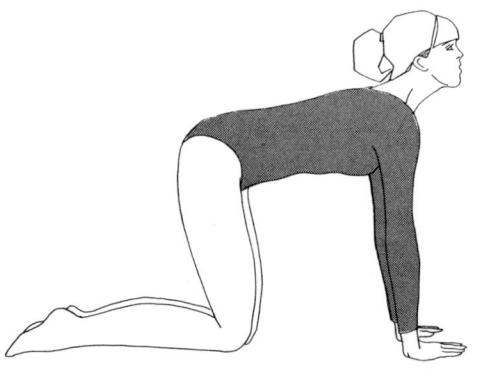

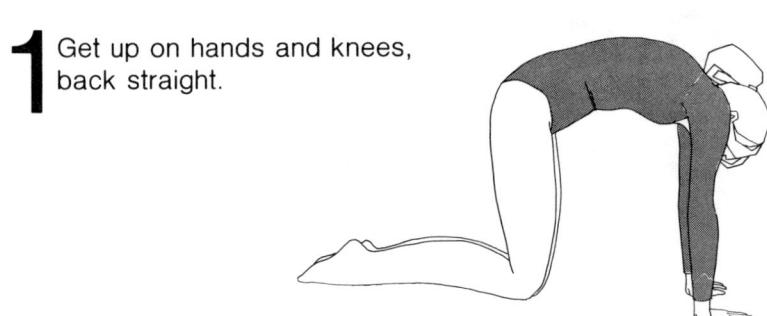

1 Get up on hands and knees, back straight.

2 Drop head, round up back as high as it will go, pulling in with abdominal muscles. Do not shift knees or hands. Hold for count of 3 or 4.

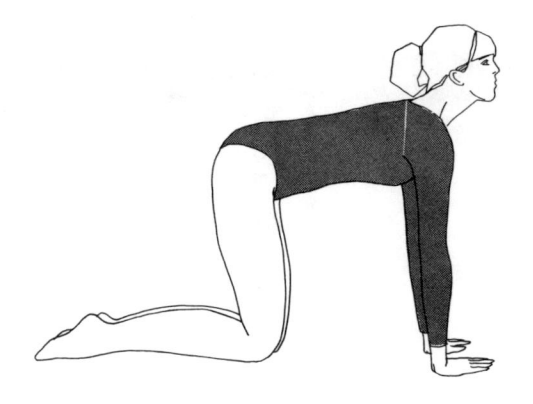

3 Lower back to position 1 and hold.
Repeat 4 times at start; aim toward 8 as capacity increases.

- **Never jerk up or down; perform movements slowly, with control.**
- **Breathe normally throughout.**

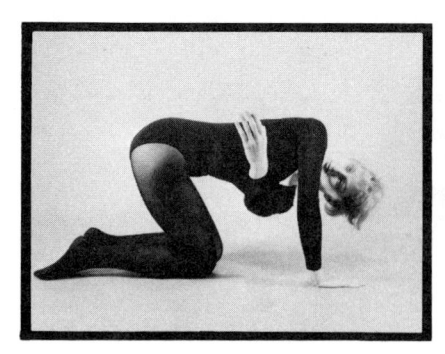

17 Angry Cat Swing

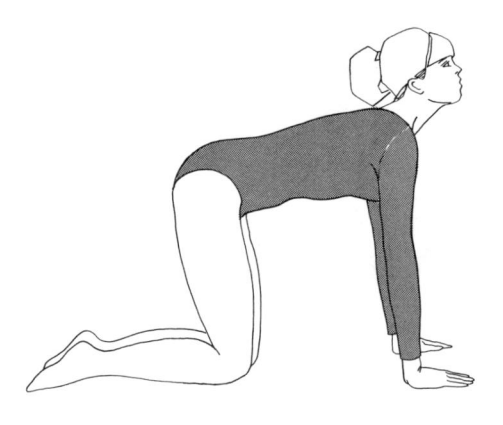

1 From position 1 of Angry Cat, shift weight to left hand, freeing right.

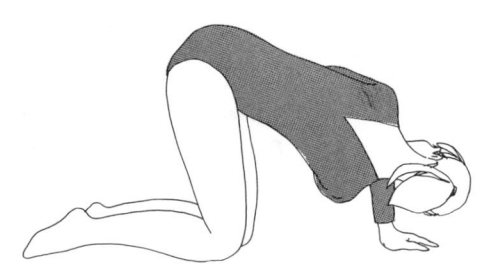

2 Twisting from waist, swing right arm under bridge made by left arm, allowing right shoulder to follow arm without forcing.

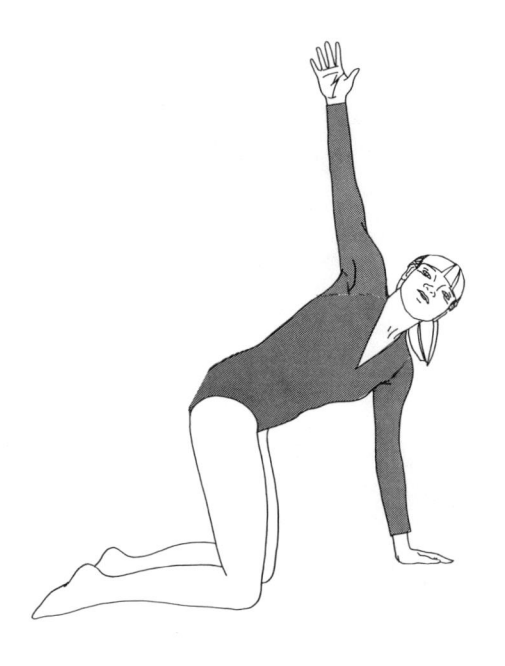

3 Swing right arm back toward right and up, looking out along raised arm.
Repeat 8 times with each arm.

- **Keep the spine as straight as possible.**
- **Try to get a full and free swing with each repeat.**

18 Leg Lift

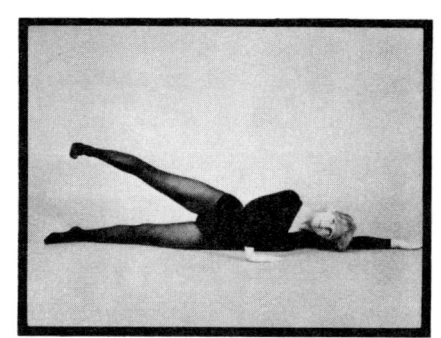

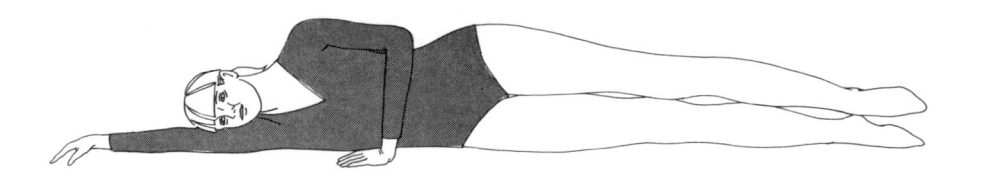

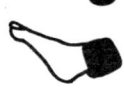

1 Lie on mat on your right side with right arm stretched up to support head; keep head, shoulders, hips, and feet in straight line. Bring left arm down in front of chest, palm flat on mat to support body and keep it from rolling forward or back.

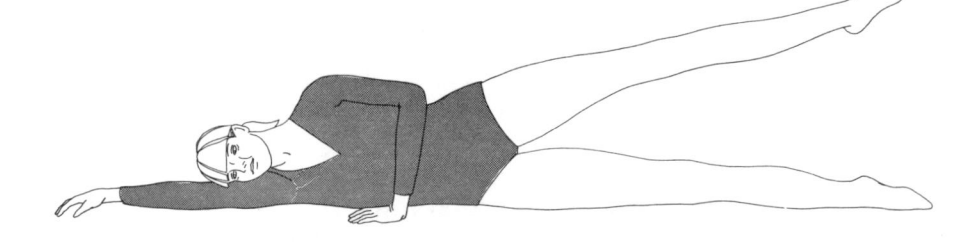

2 Point left toe and raise and lower left leg to a measured count. When the leg comes down do not permit it to touch the right leg.

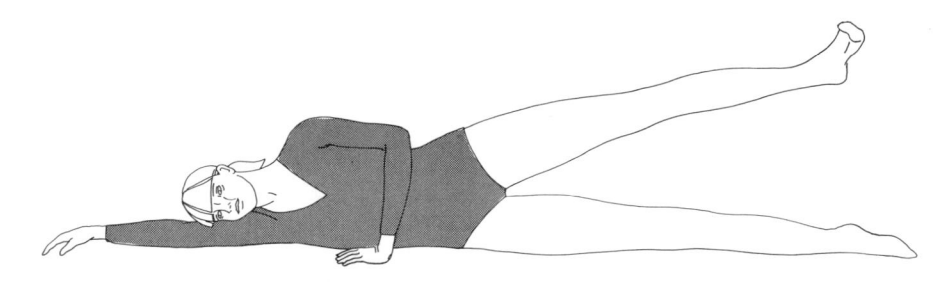

3 With foot flexed, repeat 8 times. Roll over onto left side and repeat entire routine with right leg.

Repeat 8 times with pointed toe, then repeat 8 times with foot flexed. Roll over onto left side and repeat with right leg.

- **The pointed-toe lift should be done fairly slowly; the flexed lift can be faster.**
- **Raise the leg as high as it will go without forcing, but a high lift is not the object of this exercise. It's more important to maintain the body alignment and balance.**
- **Keep both knees straight throughout.**
- **If using ankle weights, be sure to keep legs slightly forward of the body rather than in the straight line called for above. If any strain is felt on the back, stop exercise at once and do not repeat with weights.**

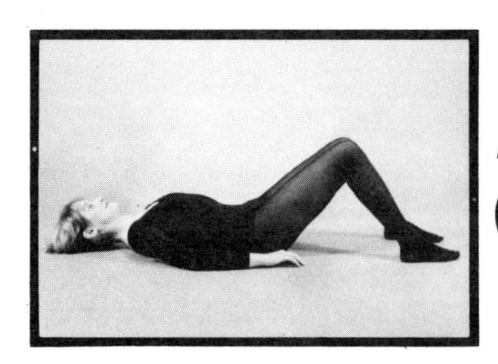

19 Abdomen Cincher

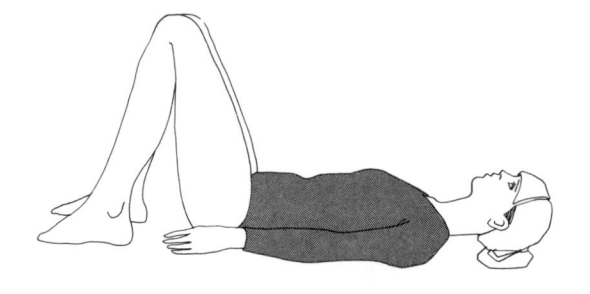

1 Lie flat on mat, arms out to sides, palms down. Bend knees up, place feet flat on mat, parallel, about shoulder-width apart, as close in toward hips as comfortable.

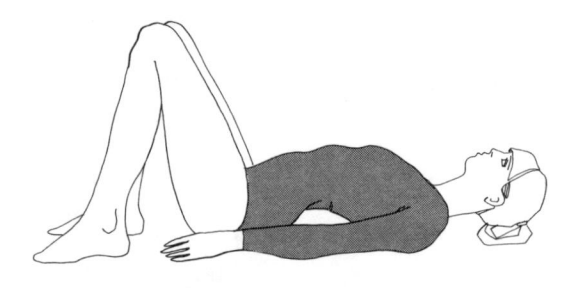

2 Arch small of back and push abdomen out as far as possible, inhaling on this motion to count of 4.

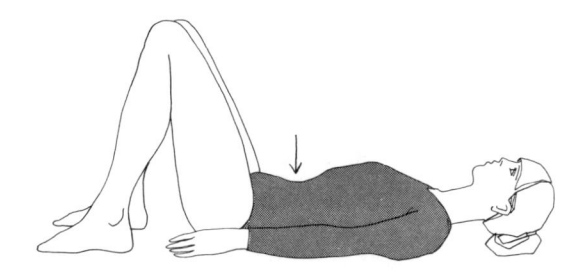

3 Exhaling, pull abdomen in, down toward mat, then press small of back hard into mat as though trying to push through floor. Count 4 slowly while continuing to pull in and down. Relax and take a few normal breaths.
Repeat 8 times.

- **Shoulders and hips should remain on the mat throughout.**

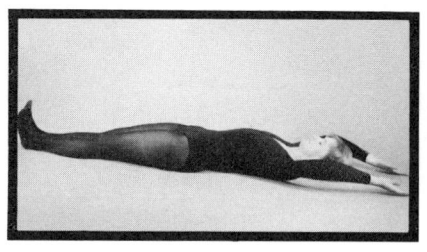

20 Refresher Stretch

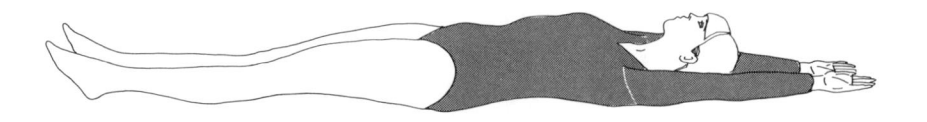

1 Stretch out on back. Toes pointed, arms up overhead.

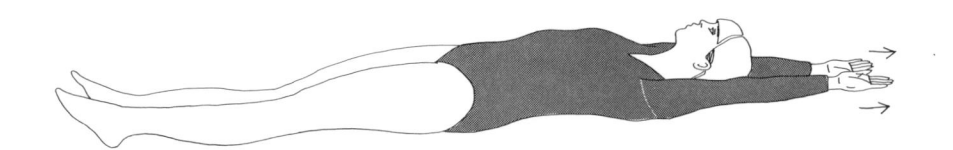

2 Push hard with arms as though pushing against a rock; relax.

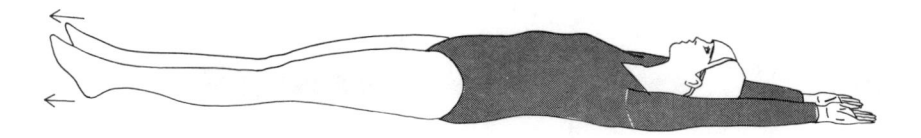

3 Push hard with legs in the same way, as though bracing them against a barrier; relax.

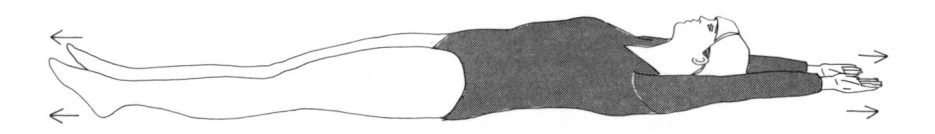

4 Push with arms and legs simultaneously, as hard as you can.

5 Hold for a few seconds, and relax.

- **Try to keep small of back against mat throughout.**

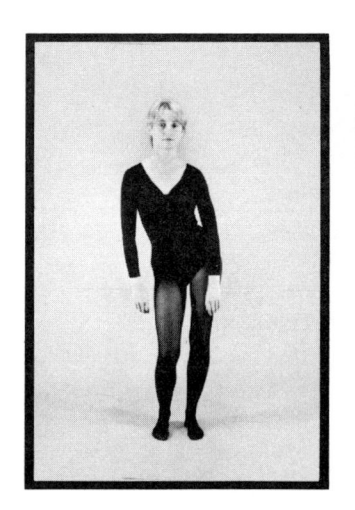

21 Hip Wiggle

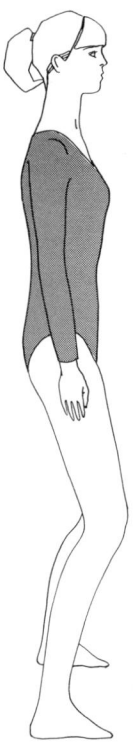

1 Stand with feet parallel, about hip-width apart, arms hanging loosely at sides. Bend knees enough to imagine you are sitting on the edge of a high stool.

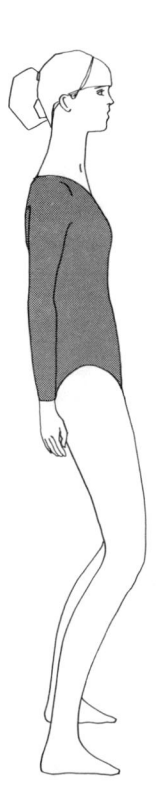

2 Start moving the hips from side to side so that each movement hits the inside of the arm on that side. Move only the hips. Repeat 6 times to each side.

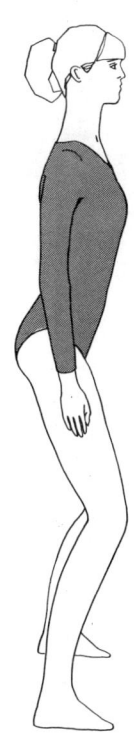

3 From the same "sitting" position, move hips forward and back. Repeat 6 times.

4 When you have the above movements under control, put them together to do a complete hula roll—forward, side, back, opposite side.
Alternating sides, repeat 6 times clockwise, 6 times counterclockwise.

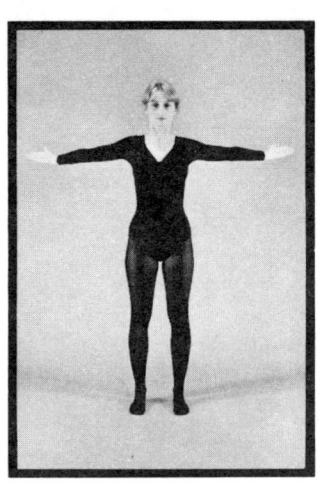

22 Upper-Arm Tightener

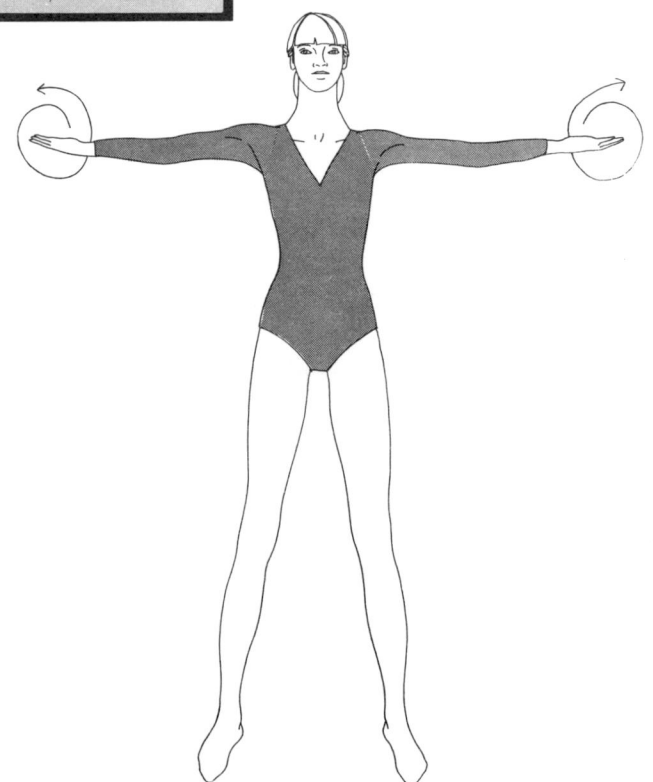

1 Stand tall, feet parallel and comfortably apart. Lift arms out sideways to shoulder level, elbows straight, palms up.

2 Moving arms only, make small circles in the air, coming forward, up, back, and around. Gradually enlarge the circles until they are beach-ball size. Do 16 circles in this direction.

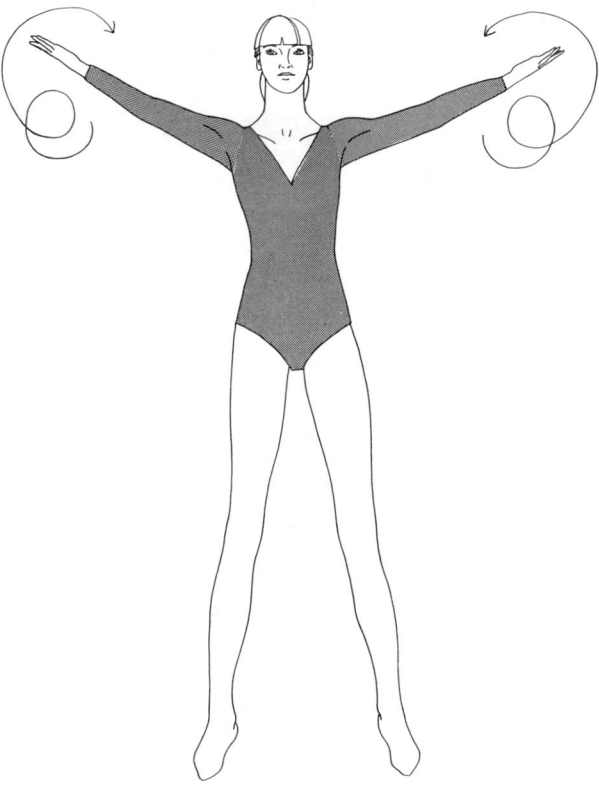

3 Reversing the direction of the arm movement (down, back, up, forward) begin with the large circle and in 16 counts bring the movement down to very small tight circles. Keep the palms facing up.

4 Roll shoulders to loosen them. Shake out arms and legs.

- **Keep arms at shoulder level and elbows straight throughout.**
- **Because of the momentum, the head will have a tendency to jut forward. Concentrate on keeping good body alignment, ears over shoulders, chest open, shoulders down, abdomen pulled in.**

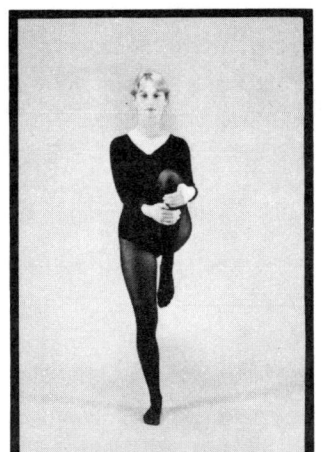

23 Thigh Stretch

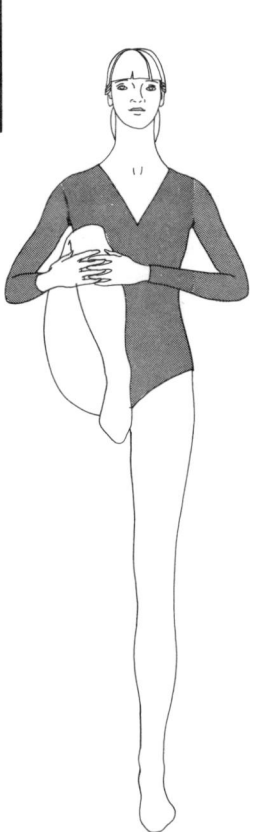

1 Stand tall. With left leg straight, bring right knee up to chest, clasping hands around knee to pull it close. Inhale on the upward motion. Hold for slow count of 4. Exhale while holding.

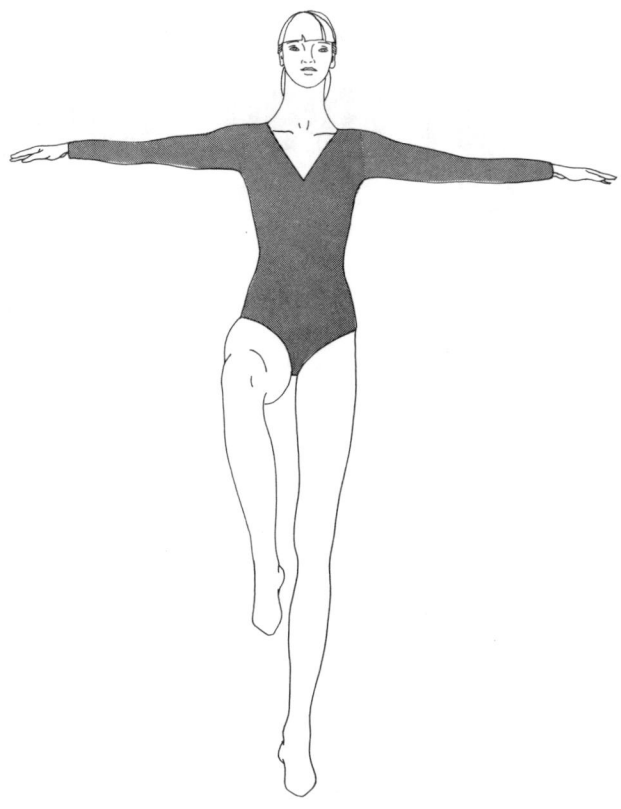

2 Lower leg, spreading arms outward. Breathe normally on this motion.

3 Repeat with left knee. Alternating legs, repeat 6 times with each leg.

- **Concentrate on posture. Don't bend the body forward to meet the knee.**
- **There will be a tendency to arch the small of the back. Remember to keep it straight, abdomen pulled in. With weights this is even more important.**

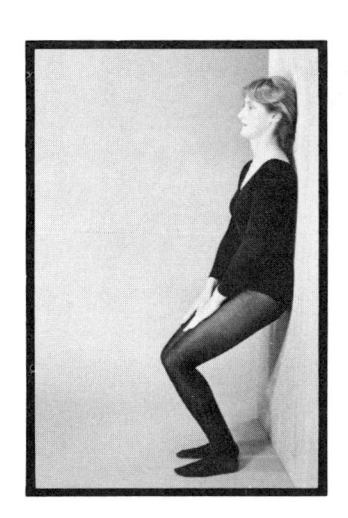

24 Thigh Tightener

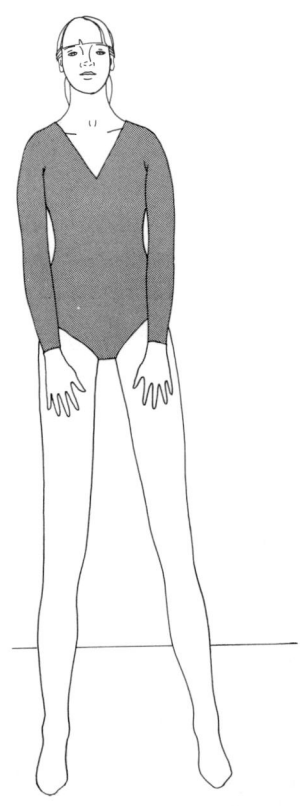

1 Stand tall with back pressed against wall, hands on hips. Move feet forward until heels are 12 to 14 inches out from wall.

2 Slide down slowly into a chair-sitting position, making sure each vertebra touches the wall as you go down. Hold this position as long as possible, at least 15 seconds for a start. The optimum count would be 90 seconds, but this is for experts. If you can bring yourself up to 30, your thighs will be tighter and trimmer in just a few weeks.

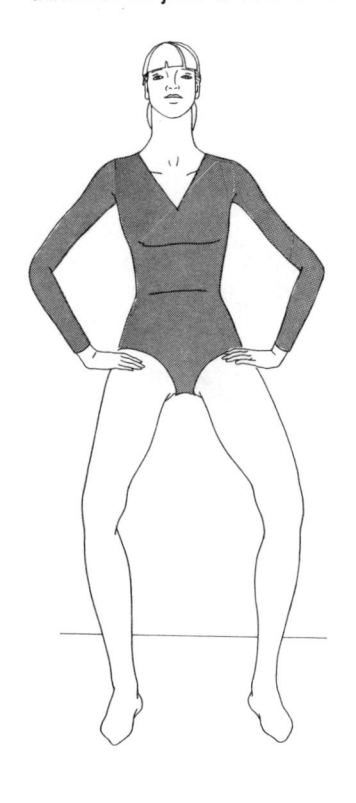

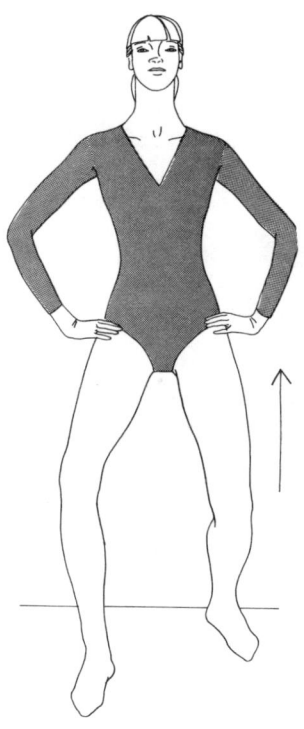

3 Recovery from this "sitting" position is important. Slide one foot back toward the wall for balance; then push back up the wall as you come down, each vertebra touching.

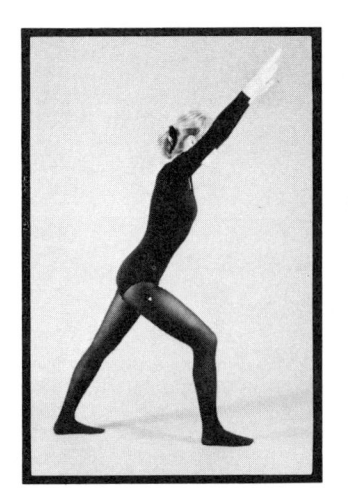

25 Lunge

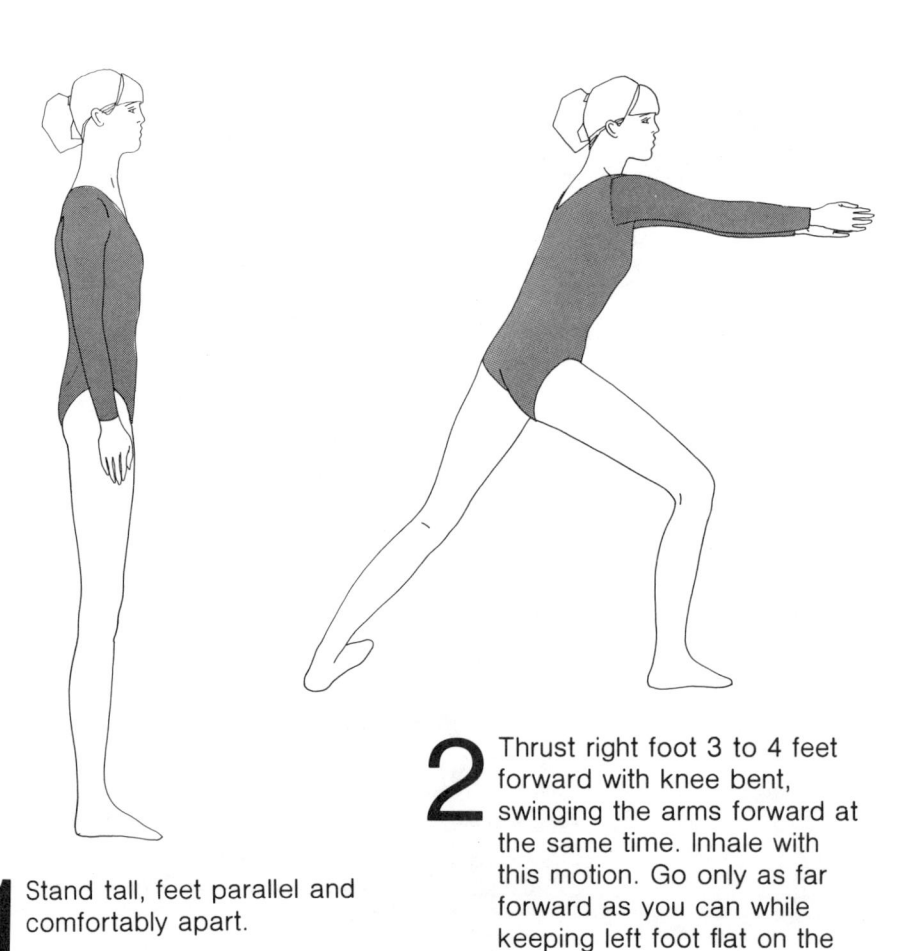

1 Stand tall, feet parallel and comfortably apart.

2 Thrust right foot 3 to 4 feet forward with knee bent, swinging the arms forward at the same time. Inhale with this motion. Go only as far forward as you can while keeping left foot flat on the floor.

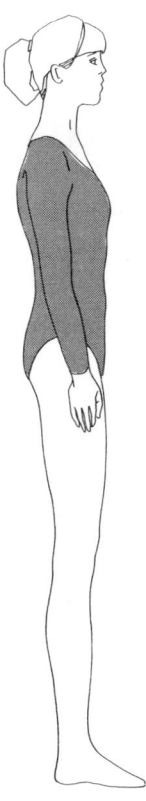

3 Pull back, dropping arms, to upright position. Exhale on this motion.

4 Repeat with left foot. Alternating sides, do 8 lunges with each foot.

- **Don't rush. Work to a measured count of your own choosing.**
- **At the peak of the lunge, the head, body, and back leg should make a diagonal line. Don't bend the head forward or thrust the chest out.**

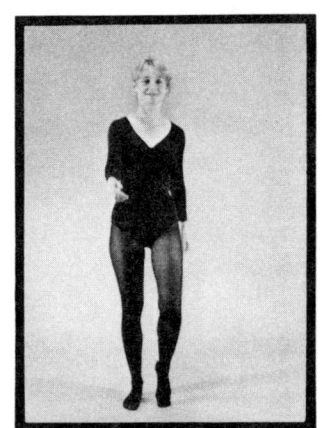

26 Jogging Down

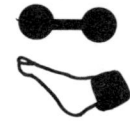

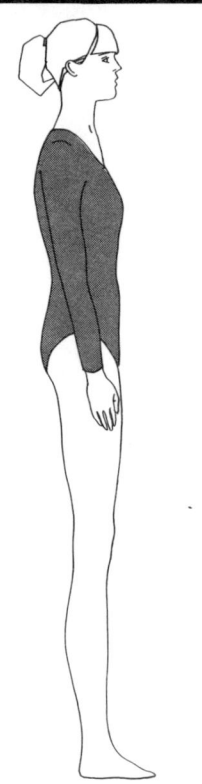

1 Stand tall, shoulders down, feet comfortably apart.

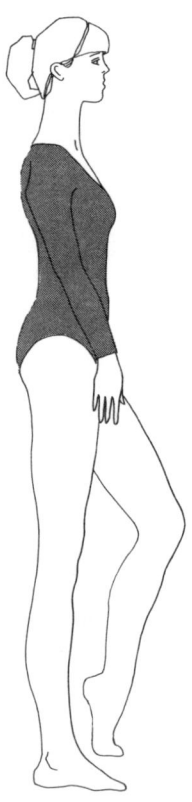

2 Roll the weight up onto the ball of one foot, then down and up onto the ball of the other foot. Keep the movement continuous and increase the pace, so that you approximate a jogging motion with the feet not actually leaving the floor.

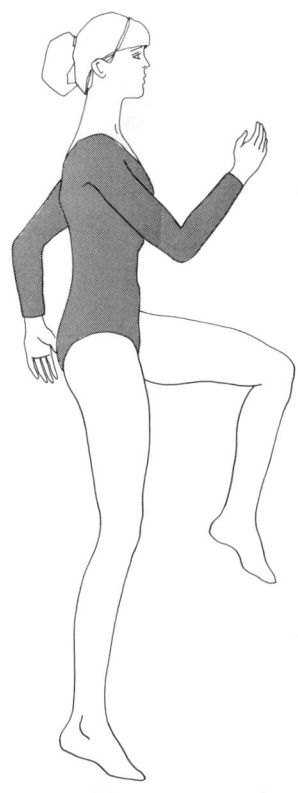

3 As you achieve momentum, move into jogging in place with the feet leaving the ground, knees coming up with each jog, arms pumping forward and back as though running. Try to continue for 1 minute at start.

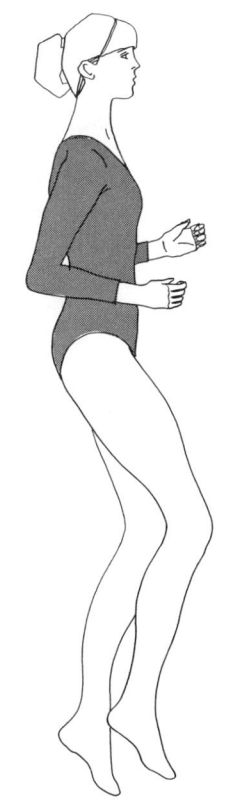

4 Very gradually, slow the pace of the jog and bring the motion back to the stationary "jog" of position 2. When the feet are no longer leaving the floor transform the movement into a walking pace and walk around the room for a minute or two. Don't collapse. Don't flop down.

- **The walk around the room is important. The heartbeat has been elevated and must be brought down slowly.**

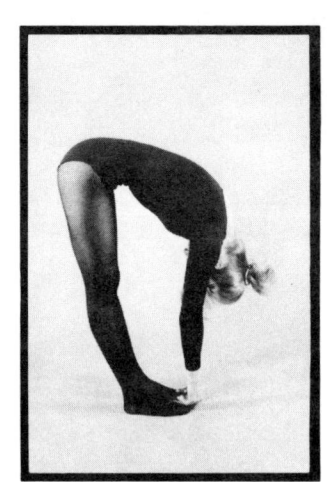

27 Rag Doll

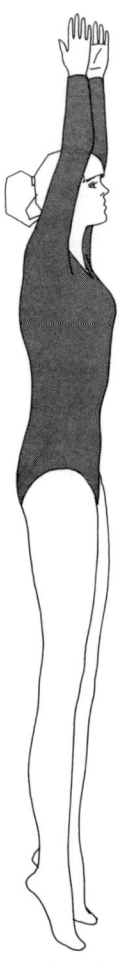

1 Standing, stetch up as far as possible, inhaling.

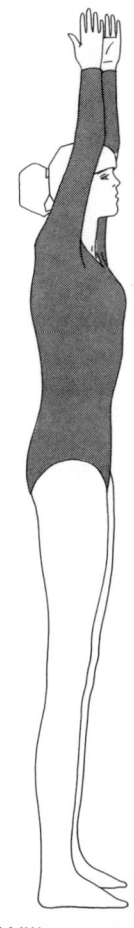

2 With arms still up, relax body, exhaling.

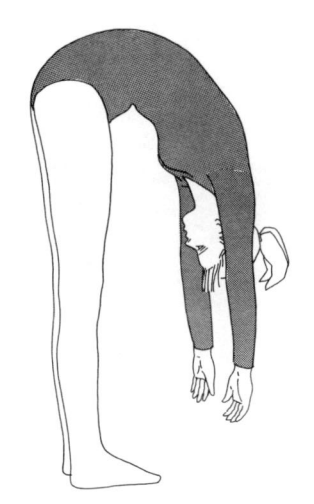

3 Flop over like a rag doll, bending from the waist, head and arms flapping loosely. Feel a good pull along spine and legs.

Chapter 4
The Emergency Shape-Up

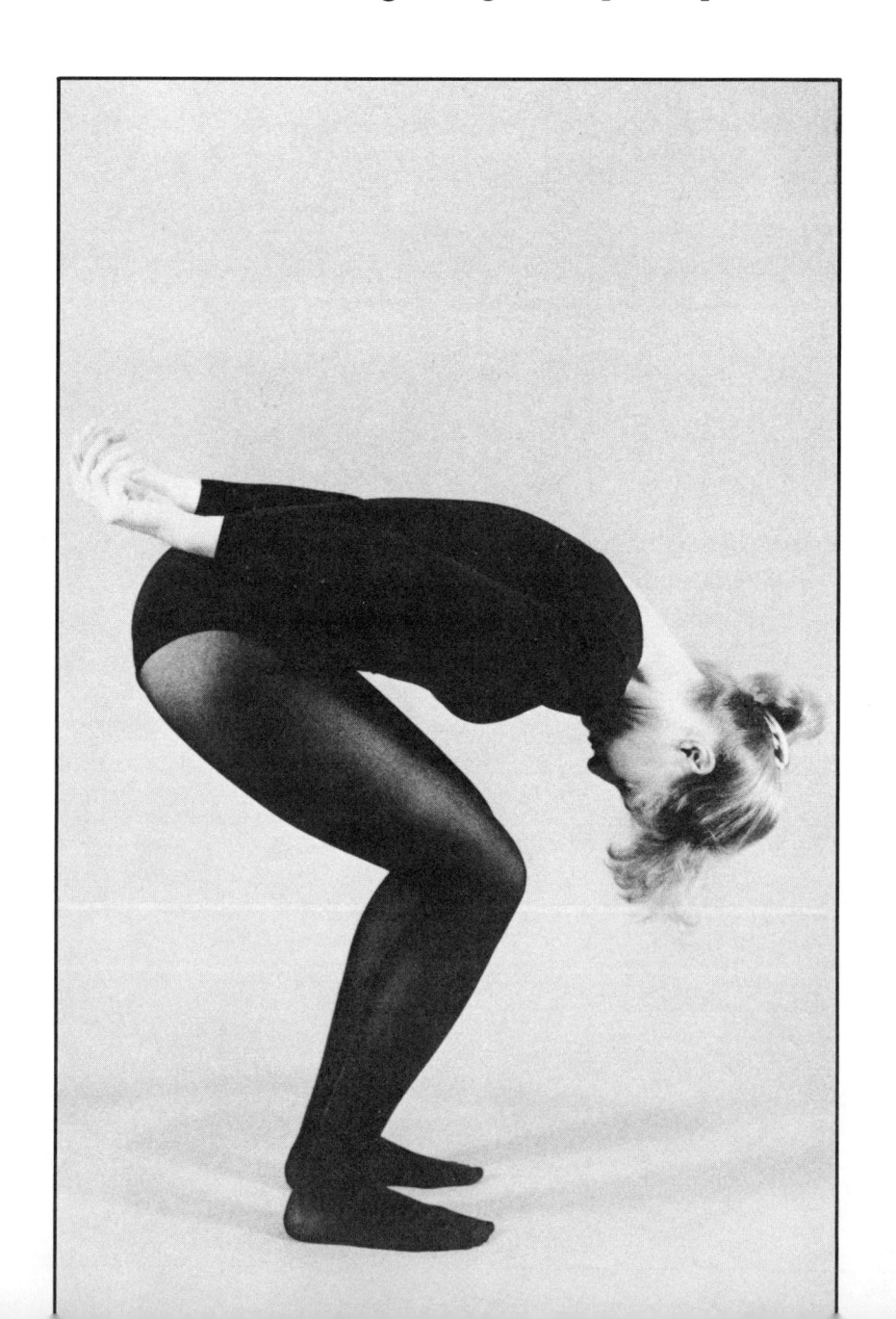

It will happen to you as it does to everyone—the day when there isn't time for a full fitness workout. Maybe there will even be a few days in a row. Do you take an all-or-nothing approach? Not if the YW experts have anything to say about it.

What they say is that you can surely grab fifteen minutes out of any twenty-four hours, and that a fifteen-minute workout is ten times better than no workout at all. To make it easy, they've organized an emergency shape-up series of exercises from Chapter 3 that can be neatly fitted into fifteen or twenty minutes.

Use this short program when the full routine isn't possible. It will keep your muscles moving, spark up your breathing and circulation, reinforce your body's memory of what stretching and flexing are all about. Above all, it will sustain your continuity and momentum, making sure you don't slide two steps back for every forward step you've worked so hard to achieve.

Remember: If you must be on short rations, at least keep the faith. It will pay off when you're once again able to work on the full routine that is the heart of this program.

Emergency Shape-up

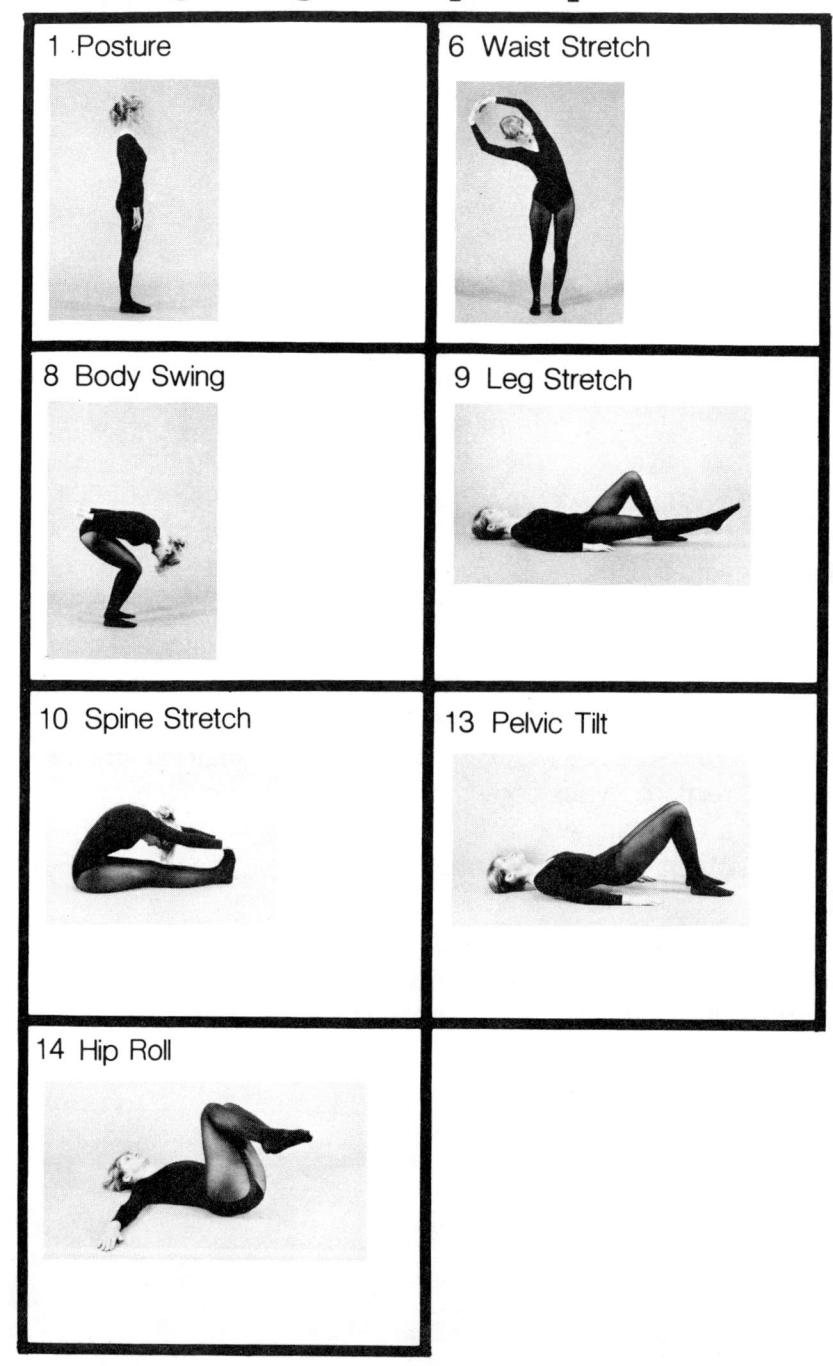

1. Posture	6 Waist Stretch
8 Body Swing	9 Leg Stretch
10 Spine Stretch	13 Pelvic Tilt
14 Hip Roll	

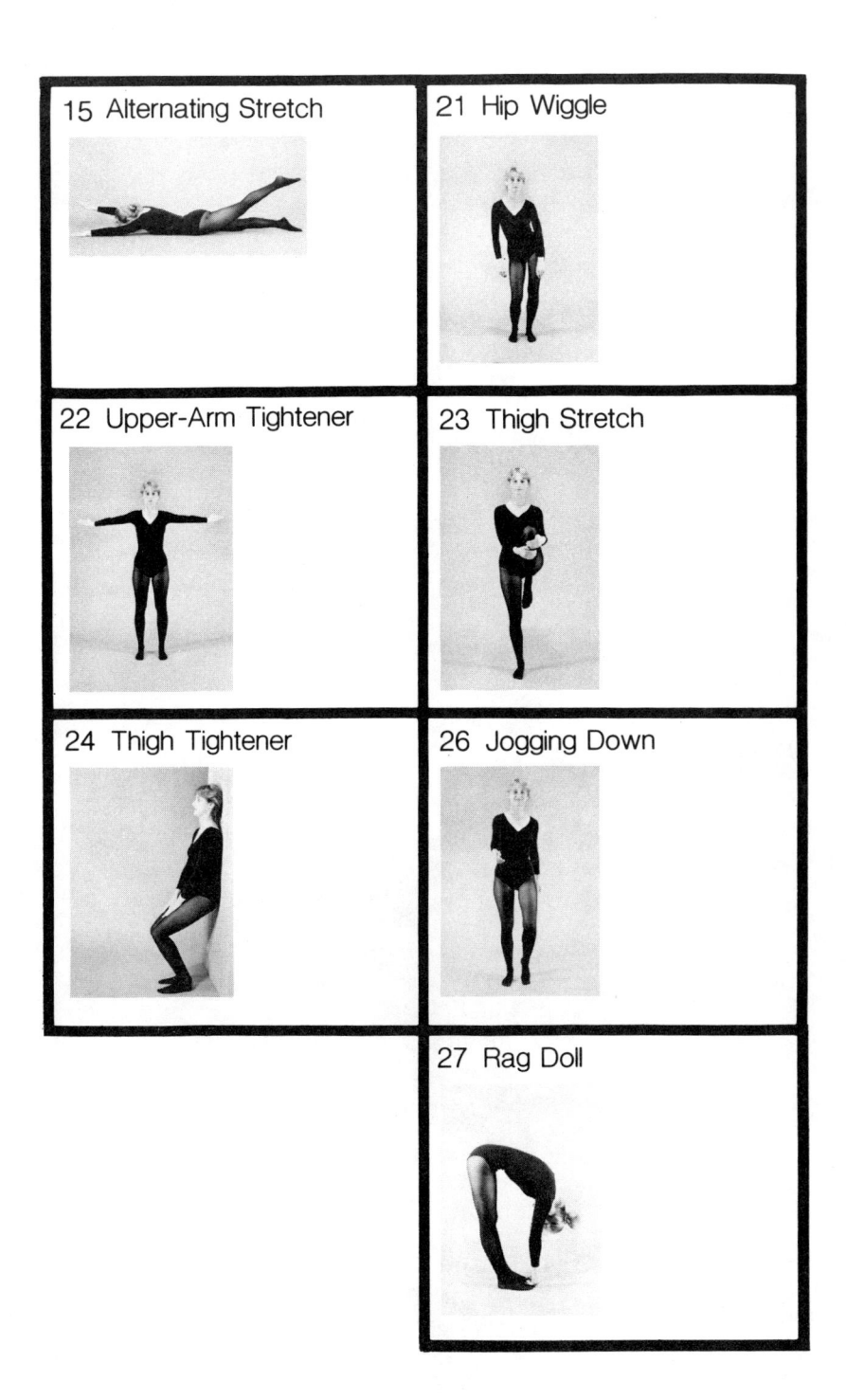

15 Alternating Stretch	21 Hip Wiggle
22 Upper-Arm Tightener	23 Thigh Stretch
24 Thigh Tightener	26 Jogging Down
	27 Rag Doll

Chapter 5
The Working Back

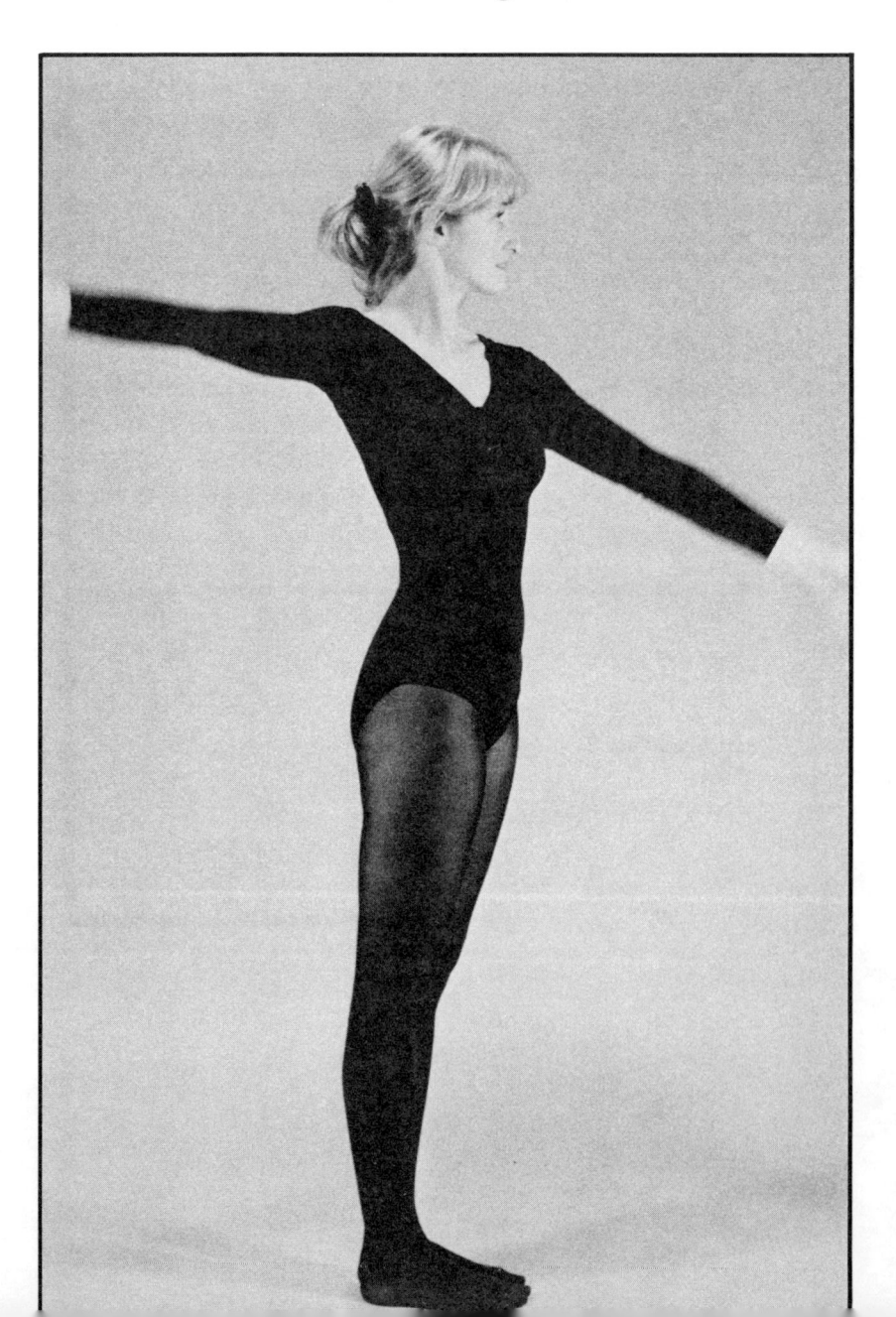

You've never been in thrall to your back. You've looked with sympathy at friends whose backs "go out." Or whose doctors diagnose slipped discs. Or who bend and can't straighten, with their backs in spasm. That's never happened to you.

You're lucky. At a conservative estimate, there are 75 million Americans who can't make that claim.

All the same, just lately there's been a difference. You're aware of your back as you never were before. Sometimes when you get up in the morning, it's uncooperative. It doesn't move fluidly; it's stiff. When you wear normally high heels you have a tendency to slip them off, or want to, long before the end of the day, not necessarily because your feet hurt but because getting off those heels eases an ache in the lumbar area. And in the evening, sometimes, the ache becomes something you have to call discomfort. Not quite pain. But there's an overwhelming wish to get off your feet with your legs up until the discomfort goes away.

In spite of your good record to date, you may be about to join the club.

This is another one of life's multitudinous nuisances that you really don't need. But according to Dr. Sonia Weber, founder of the Columbia Presbyterian Medical Center Therapeutic Exercise and Posture Clinic and doyenne of the YW's Back Care program, it's the very way most of us live that makes back trouble nearly inevitable.

More than thirty-five years of research and experience go to make up Dr. Weber's conviction that *if* we stood and moved properly, and *if* we could learn to control and defuse tension, perhaps three-quarters of our back problems would never afflict us.

The program developed by Dr. Weber for the YW's Corrective Back Care classes takes special aim against this deadly duo: poor posture and tension.

Common sense reminds us that there can certainly be other reasons for back pain and malfunction. Injury, for one—we're speaking not of serious injury, which is not something to handle with exercise, but of quite mild injury. A fall on the ice that breaks no bones, or a car accident that jolts you but from which you walk away, doesn't necessarily pop up later in life as a back problem. But it can, if your back muscles are weak, stiff, inflexible. And some back pain, of course, results from internal conditions that will not be helped by exercise and may conceivably be made worse by it.

If you're a chronic back sufferer, you and your doctor already know each other too well, so this advice is not for you. But if you're one who is just beginning to notice that things back there aren't what they were, be sensible. Tell your doctor about these exercises and have him give your back a special going-over when you have the original check-up that we've already urged as a preliminary to our basic exercises in Chapter 3.

Posture

On page 54 we explained how to organize your body into the upright, balanced structure it's meant to be. With the head supported by the tower of cervical vertebrae and the strong pelvic girdle and legs bearing the weight of the torso, the body moves and works so that each muscle involved is doing the job it was designed for—provided it's strong enough to do so. When the bony framework is out of balance, it's easy enough to see that entire systems of muscles are forced to do what they are neither structured nor located to do, while other muscles go unused. The strained muscles become sore, even torn; the neglected muscles stiffen, lose tone, and gradually lose their capacity to respond even when called on. It becomes a circular syndrome: poor posture and body use weaken the muscles, and as the muscles become weaker, it becomes harder for them to support the bones in good alignment.

If your back has only lately begun to complain, perhaps it's because your posture abuses have been very minor ones, which take a longer time to show up in damage. But it's also true that as we grow older our tissues tend to grow less flexible; our hormonal balance changes, the synovial fluid that "oils" the joints diminishes somewhat, and the spinal discs gradually come to contain more cartilage and less gelatinous material. The vertebrae cannot slide on the disc as freely as before, and the discs do not cushion against friction or injury. In other words, our backs are stiffer, and sudden or unusual movement is more likely to cause trouble. Add to this those stiffened muscles, and it's a wonder that any one of us escapes an aching back.

If you refer back to Chapter 2, you'll see which of the back muscles are of chief concern in this section: the sternocleidomastoid of the neck, the trapezius and the powerful latissimus dorsi, and the three sections of the deep muscle group called the sacrospinalis, which, taken together, support almost the whole length of the spine and are instrumental in holding it erect and giving it its backward, forward, and side-to-side mobility. It's obvious that when these muscles weaken, back problems must follow.

However, what's curious about the back—and vital in helping us realize how dynamically the body operates as a total entity and not a collection of independent parts—is that much of what keeps your back in shape actually happens at the front of your body. Check back to page 28, and you'll be reminded that a lot of your back's strength is supported by the muscles that span your abdominal area from ribs to pelvis. Chiefly, these are: external or descending obliques, internal or ascending obliques, transversus and rectus abdominis.

These muscles do not lie side by side, but are constructed in three layers, one more or less behind the other: the externals outermost, the internals behind them, the transversus beneath, and all of them forming a sort of sheath for the rectus abdominis. At various points they are attached to the lower eight ribs and to the hipbone and other parts of the pelvic girdle, and to muscles in the lower back. Because of this layered arrangement, and because their fibers run in different directions—some from top to bottom, some from bottom to top, some from back to front—this complex works together to create a "corset" which keeps the abdomen strong and flat, allowing the back muscles to concentrate on supporting the spine.

But permit the abdominals to weaken, and everything literally goes to pot, and worse. They pull on the spinal muscles, weakening them in turn. Gradually—even not so gradually—the softer internal abdominal organs surge and swell forward, laying an even heavier load on the "corset" as it becomes progressively less able to cope. Unless help arrives in the form of corrective, strengthening exercise, the cycle feeds on itself and we have a miserably typical picture: exaggerated inward-curving lumbar region, potbelly, shoulders rounding forward.

Back pain is only part of the price we pay for this kind of body mismanagement. The weakening of the abdominals means that they cannot exert enough pressure on the internal organs to do what they were designed to do. Digestion becomes impaired and elimination sluggish and haphazard.

Tension

According to Webster's Dictionary, one meaning of tension is: "a state of psychic unrest often with signs of physiologic stress." And another: "the condition of being stretched to stiffness."

Taken together, the two are a complete formula for a good part of your back problem, one touching on the cause, the second (when translated into muscle terms) on a major effect. Remember, too, that every muscle thus "tensed" is partnered by its opposing muscle, constricted into prolonged, unnatural immobility. Now visualize your spine: see the sternocleidomastoid of the neck, or the long sacrospinalis that supports almost the whole length of the spine, being asked to bend or make any quick movement while in this condition, and you'll better understand why tension is so high on the Back Care enemies list.

Granted, tension is a symptom. But this book is not about to take on the causes, fundamental though they may be. In a general sense, we all have a pretty good idea what they are, just from getting up every morning and going out into the world.

Learning to handle these tensions is another subject entirely. The "psychic unrest" they create cannot be our problem here. The best we can do is deal with their physiological fallout.

It's against this physiologic stress that our back-care exercises are designed to work. They will unravel those knots, smooth out the kinks, get muscles and tendons and joints functioning smoothly and strongly again. Do them well, and you should see improvement in a few weeks. More important, you will be learning a powerful defense against any back threats in your future.

Ground Rules For Back Care Exercises

As with the exercises in Chapter 3, you can improve your results by keeping in mind a few general rules.

• Work slowly. In these exercises the stretch-and-hold is particularly important. Get the most stretch possible out of each movement.

• Move smoothly. Never jerk into action.

• Be aware of your breathing. Try to learn to coordinate breathing with movement—breathing in on the action, out on the release.

• Stop often between exercises if you feel tired or strained and relax in the Cat Rest position (page 144). Or repeat the Constructive Relaxation exercise (page 120).

• If during any exercise you feel any degree of pain, stop at once and rest. Resume with an exercise that works a different part of the body. Under no circumstances should you continue working if pain persists or returns

A SPECIAL QUICK MUSCLE-ADEQUACY TEST

Before you begin the back exercises, it is important that you determine the present condition of your body muscles.

This six-part test was devised by the noted back specialist Dr. Hans Kraus and by Dr. Sonia Weber, creator of the YW's back care program. The test is used internationally to gauge muscular adequacy.

In looking over the test, note that it is suggested you have someone at hand to help.

Most important: these are not exercises. They are simply tests to determine the present state of your muscles. Chances are you will have trouble with some or all of them. Do not strain to achieve maximum results. Do only as much as is comfortable. Then spend as much time as you can on the exercises in this chapter and retest yourself at two- or three-week intervals. If you're working properly, you should find steady improvement.

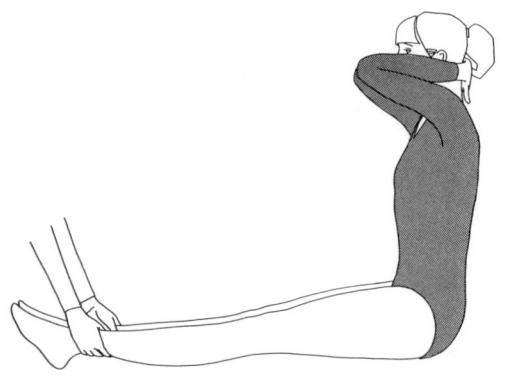

1 Lie flat on back, hands clasped behind neck, legs straight out and feet anchored in place. One way to do this is to get someone to hold them for you; failing that, hook them beneath a heavy piece of furniture. Then roll up into sitting position. You pass if you can accomplish one sit-up. This tests the *hip flexors* and the *abdominals*.

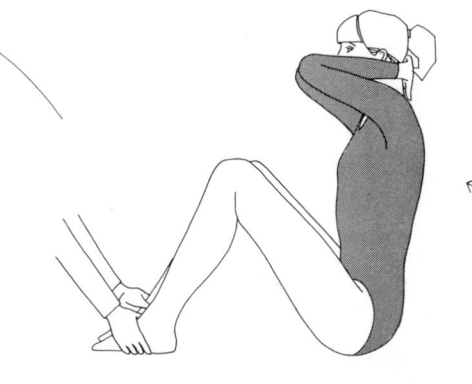

2 Lie flat on back, hands clasped behind neck, knees in tent position but with feet anchored as in Test 1. Roll up into sitting position. This tests the *abdominals*.

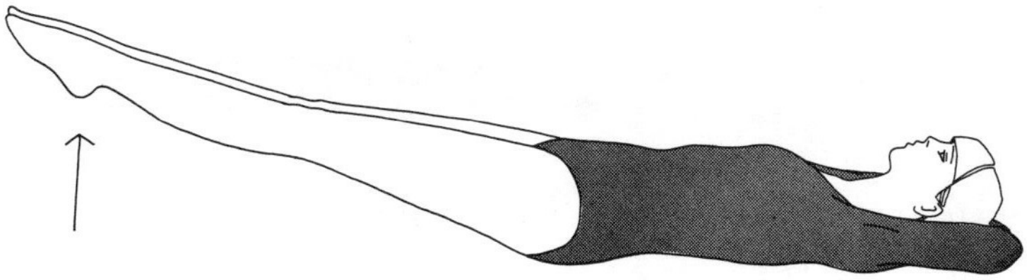

3 Lie flat on back, hands clasped behind head, legs straight out. Keeping everything else in place, raise the legs together to about 10 inches above the floor. Hold for 10 seconds. This tests the *Flexors*.

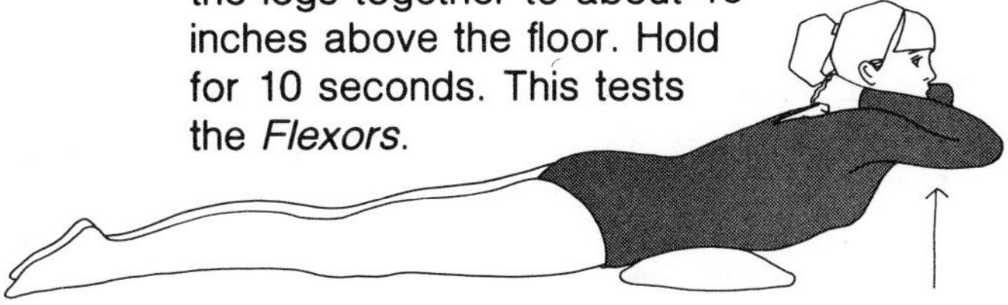

4 For this and for Test 5 which follows, you are better off working with a partner. Lie face down with a pillow under the abdomen, hands clasped behind neck.
Lift the upper part of your body and hold it steady for 10 seconds. This tests *upper back muscles*.

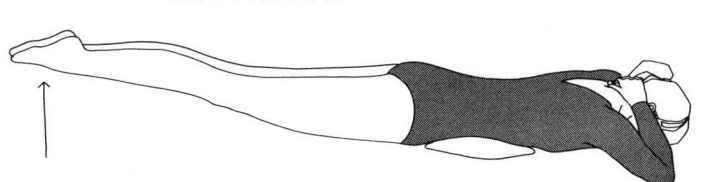

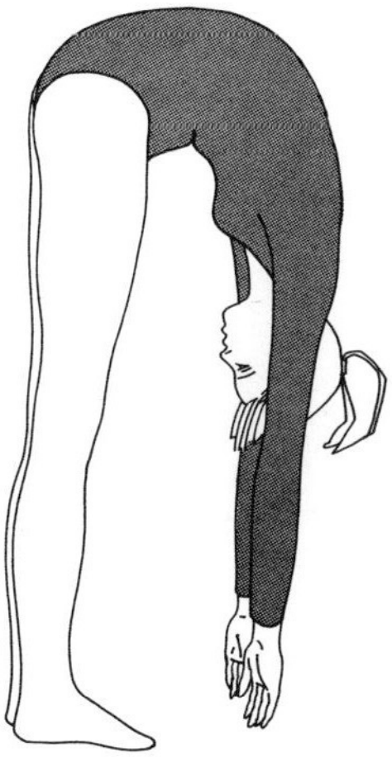

5 Lie face down, pillow under abdomen, hands clasped behind neck. Have your partner hold your upper back steady at shoulders and hips, as shown. Raise the legs from the hips, straight and together, and hold for 10 seconds. This tests *lower back muscles*.

6 Stand straight, feet together, arms at sides. Relax and bend over, trying to touch the floor with your fingertips without bending your knees. This tests tension and flexibility in *back muscles* and *hamstrings*.

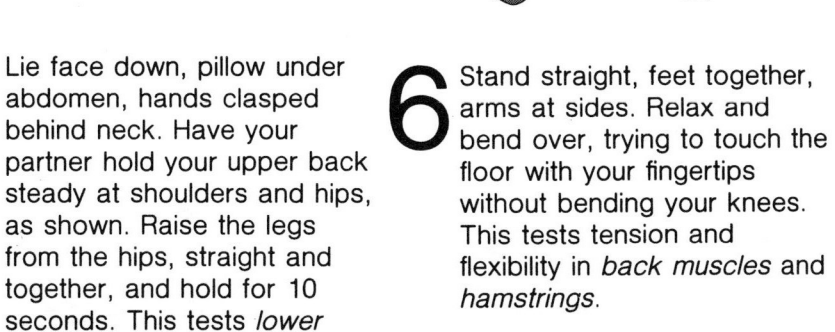

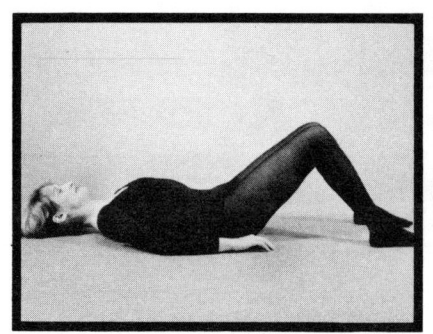

1 Constructive Relaxation

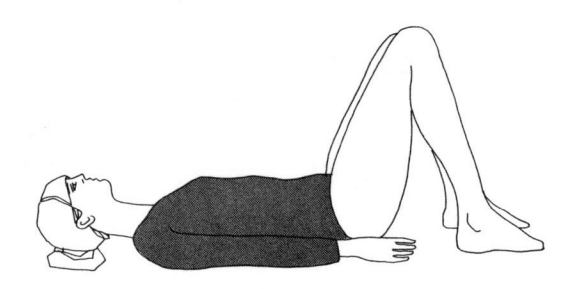

1 Lie on back in "tent" position: knees up, feet flat on mat, hip-width apart. Keep chin as close to front of neck as possible. In the exercises that follow, this is what is meant when you are asked to take the tent position.

2 Allow knees to rest against one another, completely relaxed.

3 Arms lie along sides, relaxed.

4 Feel the whole length of your back against the mat. Listen to it; be aware of it, but without tension. Do not force your back down into the mat; as your back muscles release you will feel more of your back against the mat. Let it happen.

5 Then go on to investigate your body from top to toes. Feel each part and each member. You are looking for tension spots. When you find them, allow them to relax. Don't forget shoulders, back of neck, throat, jaw, mouth, tongue, abdomen, even fingers and toes.

6 When genuinely relaxed, your body will feel heavy. Feel the weight. Think of your heavy body as sinking through the floor.

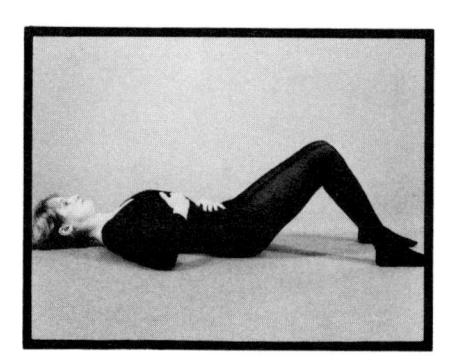

2 Breathing Drill

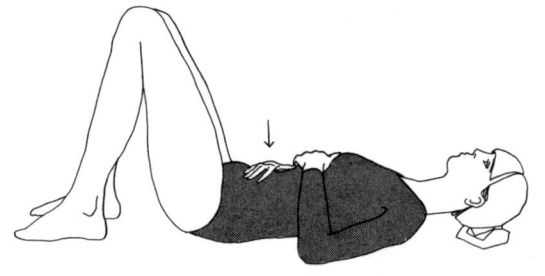

1 Lie on back in tent position. Place one hand on the ribs and the other on the abdomen so that you can feel yourself breathing.

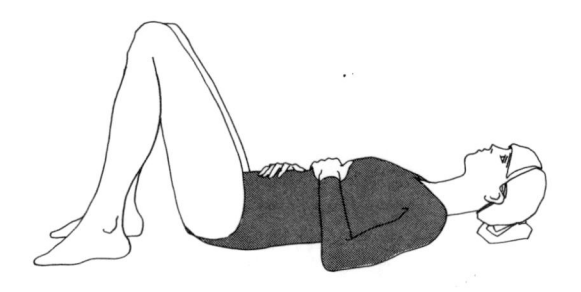

2 Take a deep, full breath in through the nose. Pull it all the way into the abdomen, allowing the chest, abdomen, and back to expand simultaneously. Feel the process under your hands.

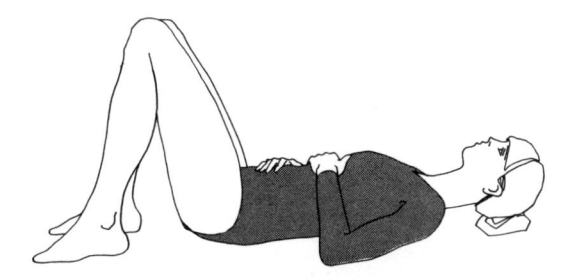

3 Push the breath completely out through the mouth with an audible exhalation.

4 Take a few normal breaths. Repeat 4 times.

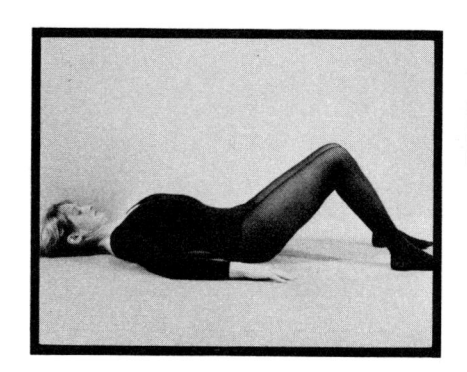

3 Neck Stretch

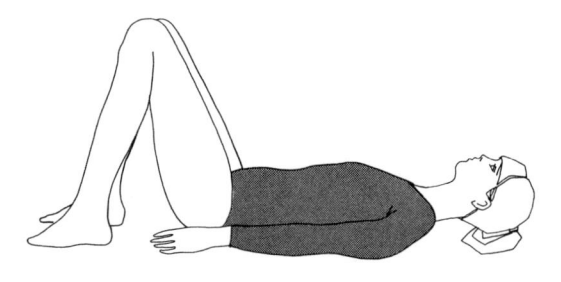

1 Lie on back in tent position. Tuck chin toward front of neck.

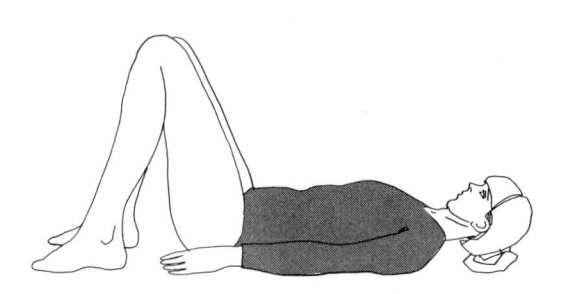

2 Without raising head, stretch back of neck.

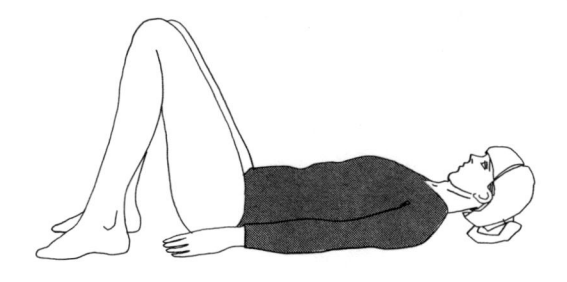

3 Hold the stretch for a slow count of 4.

4 Release.

Repeat 3 to 4 times.

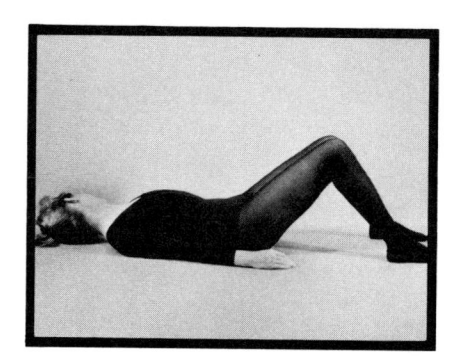

4 Head Roll

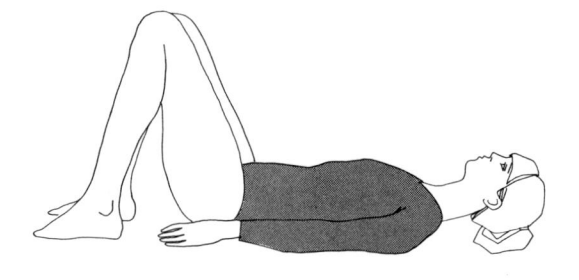

1 Lie on back in tent position.

2 Feel the weight of your head.

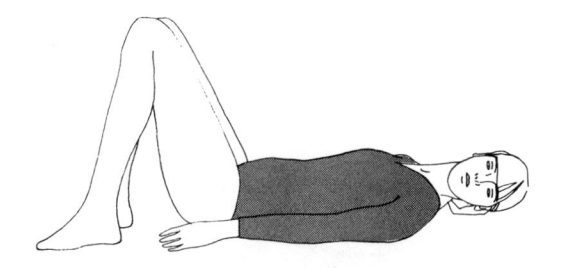

3 Let head roll to the right, back to center, to the left, back to center.

Repeat until neck feels relaxed.

- **Don't push the head. Let it roll of its own weight.**

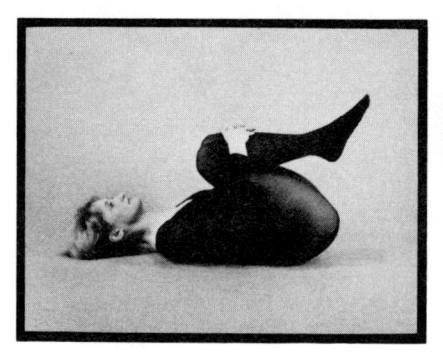

5 Low Back Stretch

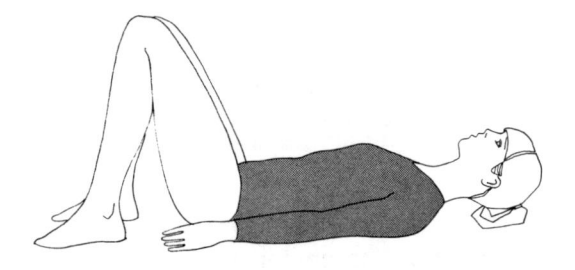

1 Lie on back in tent position. Bring knees to chest.

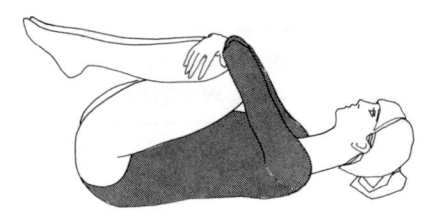

2 Wrap arms around knees, pulling them closer. Hold for count of 12.

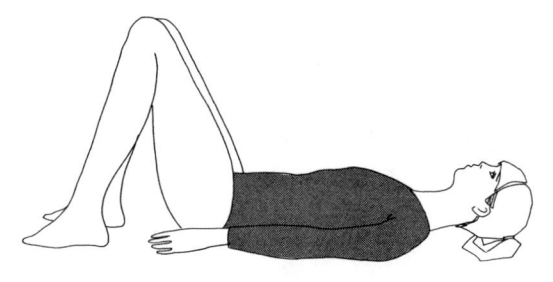

3 Return to tent position.

Repeat 4 times.

- **Don't allow your head to come up off the mat as you pull your knees closer.**

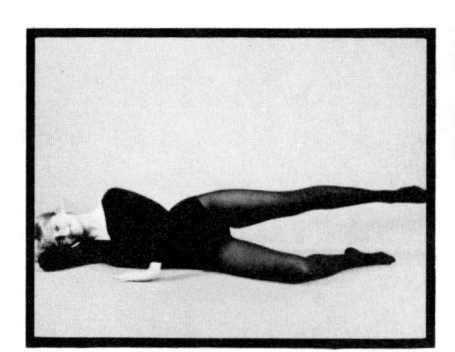

6 Leg Slide

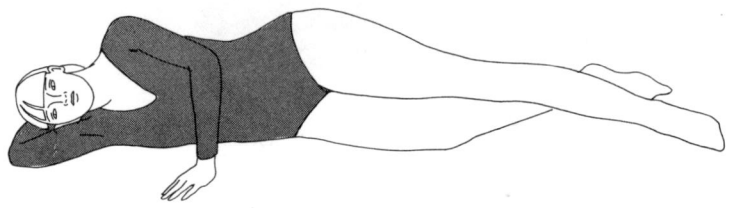

1 Stretch out on mat, lying on right side. Fold the right arm back so that it makes a rest for the head. Place the left palm on the mat in front of the body for support. Bend the right leg slightly so that the left leg can lie on it relaxed. Check position. Head and torso should lie in a straight line. Left shoulder and hip should point toward the ceiling, not lean either forward or back.

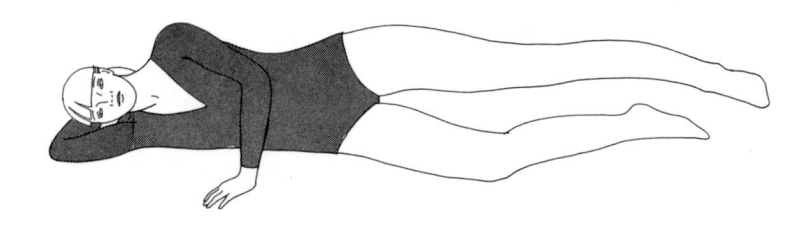

2 Stretch left leg straight down and lift it to hip height.

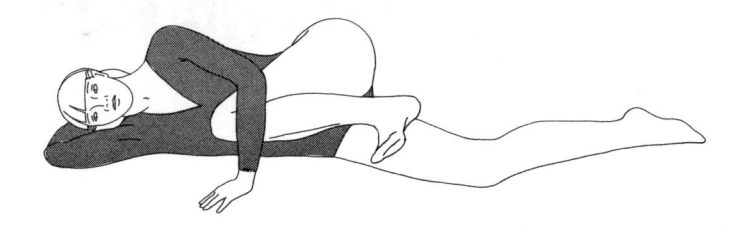

3 Draw left knee toward chest, allowing lower back to curve. Keep the movement at hip height.

4 Stretch left leg back down as in position 2. Hold briefly.

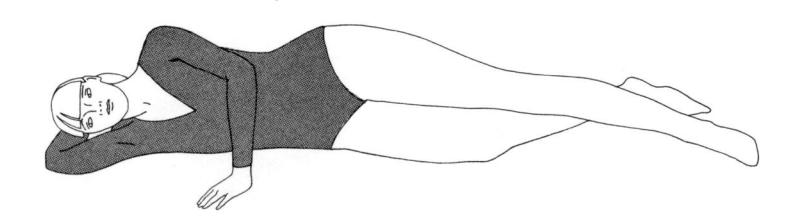

5 Release hold, allow leg to drop back to resting position as in position 1.

Repeat 3 times. Then roll over onto left side, repeat 3 times with right leg.

- **The curve of the lower back is important in this exercise, but don't allow your head to push forward as you curve the back.**

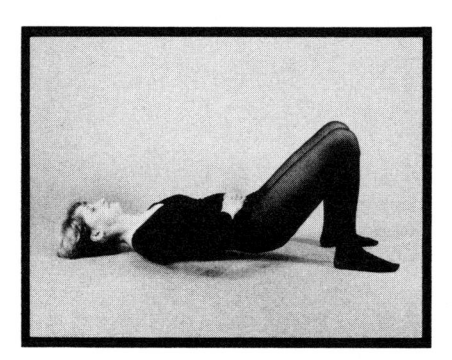

7 Pelvic Rock

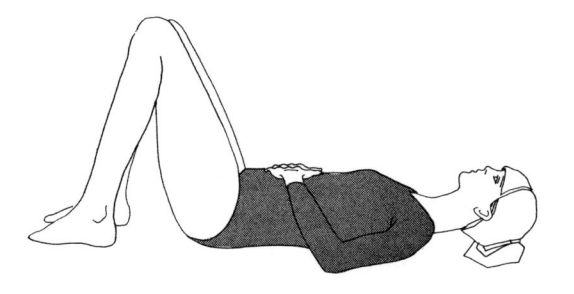

1 From side-lying position of Exercise 6, roll onto back in tent position.

2 Place hands on abdominal area to feel how the muscles work as the exercise progresses.

3 Press the small of the back into the mat.

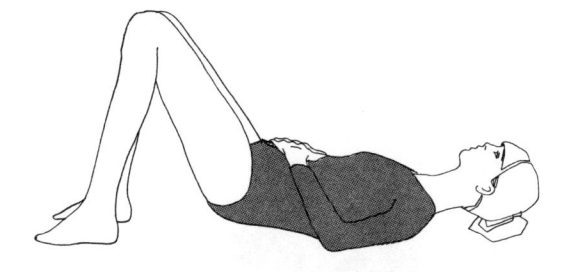

4 Gently tighten the buttocks so that the tailbone curls slightly up off the mat, no more than 1 inch.

5 Hold; release; roll down.

Repeat 4 times.

• **Don't strive for height in this rock. The purpose here is to round and stretch the lower back.**

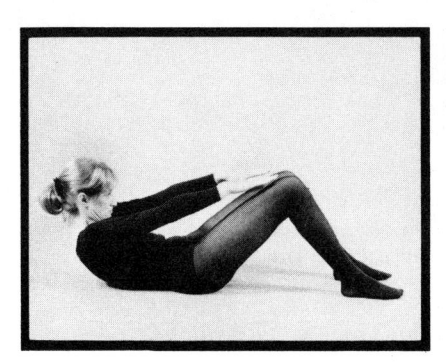

8 Curl-Up Progression

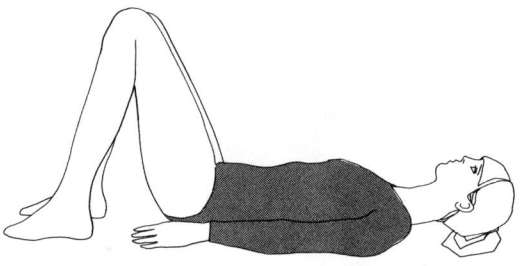

1 Lie on back in tent position.

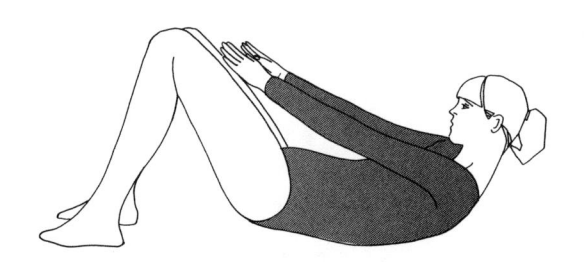

2 Tighten buttocks, bring tailbone up slightly in pelvic rock as in Exercise 7. Raise arms toward knees. Simultaneously bring head up to look at knees.

3 Lower head back to mat; release pelvic rock. Repeat 4 times.

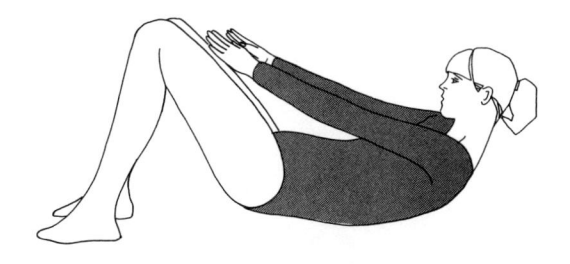

4 Repeat pelvic rock and head-raising, but this time roll head up until shoulder blades leave the mat. Hold briefly.

5 Roll down, release pelvic rock. Repeat 4 times.

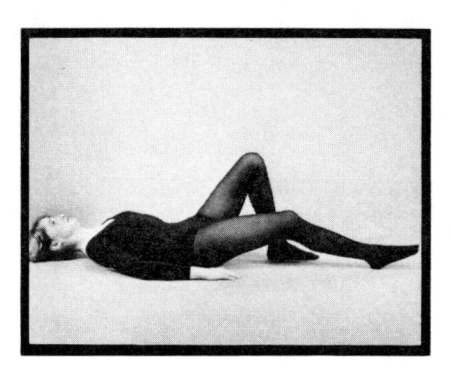

9 Hip-Thigh Stretch

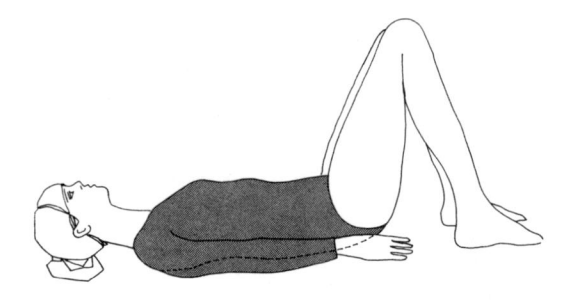

1 Lie on back in tent position. Do slight pelvic rock to pull small of back against floor.

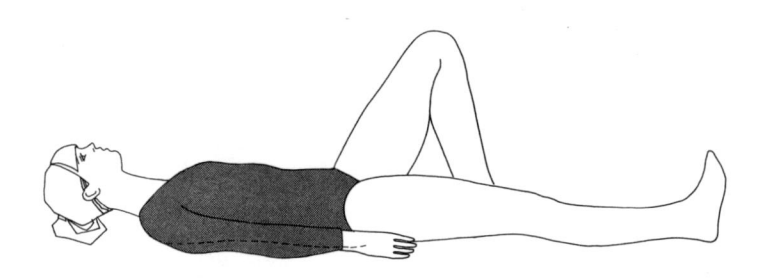

2 Holding small of back against floor, flex right foot and slide right leg down along mat slowly until it is straight *or* until the back starts to come off the mat.

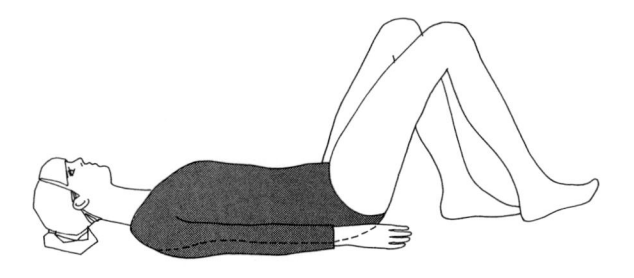

3 Deepen the pelvic rock and draw the right leg back to starting position.
Alternating legs, do 4 stretches with each leg.

• **The object here is to get as much stretch as possible into the front of the thigh and the hip while the back remains anchored to the mat. Stretch the leg out only as far as you can while keeping the back down.**

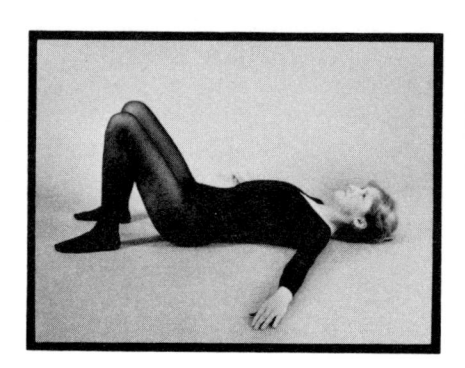

10 Hamstring Stretch

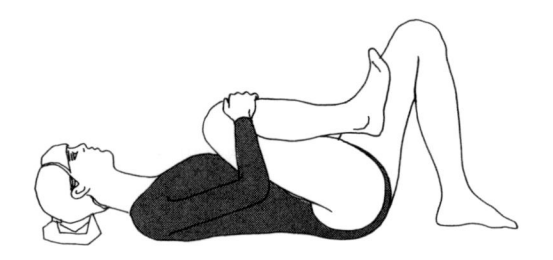

1 Lie on back in tent position. Bring right knee up toward chest, clasping hands around knee to pull it closer to chest. Flex right foot.

2 Straighten leg to point toward ceiling, sliding hands around to back of leg to support it. Point right toe.

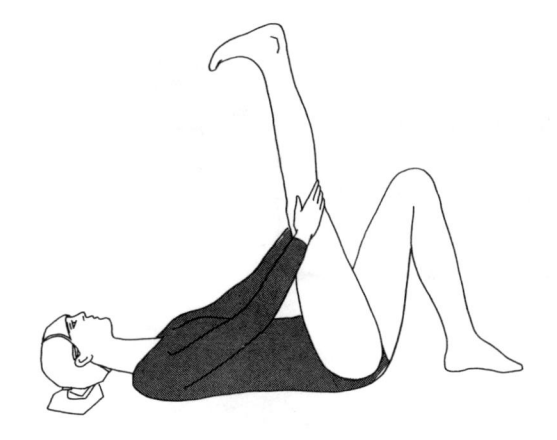

3 With leg stretched up, point right toe, then flex foot again.

4 Keeping foot flexed, bend right knee back toward chest.

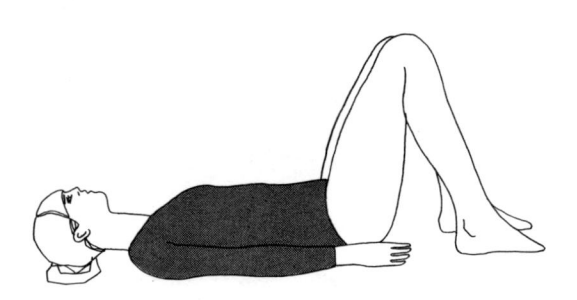

5 Return to tent position.

Alternating legs, repeat 6 times with each leg.

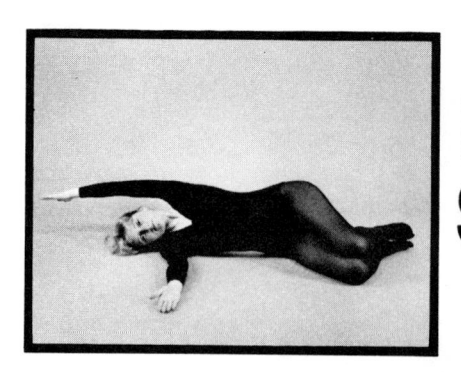

11 Pectoral Stretch

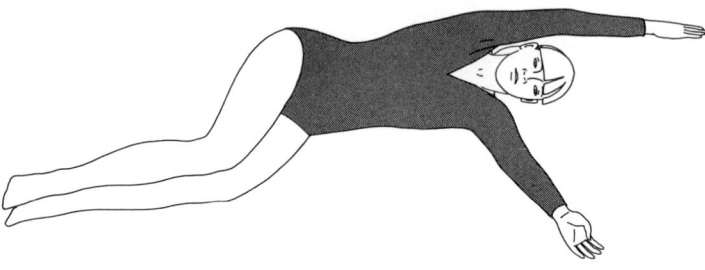

1 Lie on side, head and torso in line.
Bend knees up so that top leg rests relaxed on lower leg.

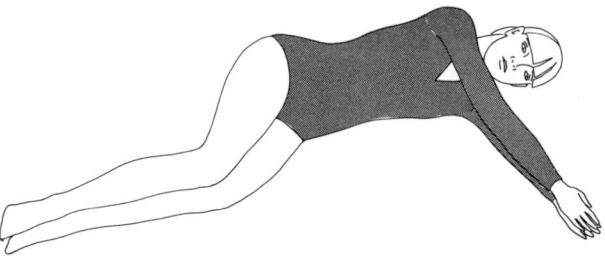

2 Extend both arms out together so that they lie relaxed on the mat at right angles to the body.

- **Keep head and shoulders loose. The purpose here is to get the widest possible stretch of the pectoral area.**
- **Keep the body and knees in their original position.**

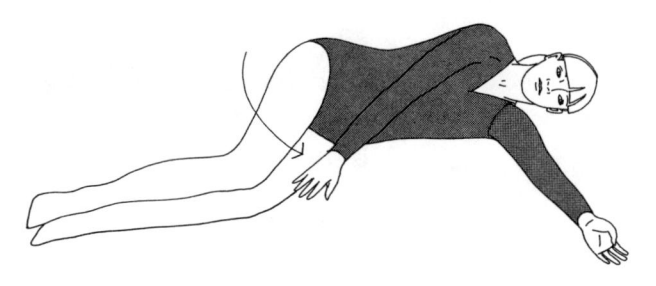

3 Raise the top arm slightly. Keeping it close to the body, move it over the head, down the back, across the body, and up forward to its original position—in other words, you are drawing a circle more or less parallel to the floor.

4 As the arm moves, allow the head and shoulder to move with it.

Repeat 4 times. Reverse direction, repeat 4 times. Roll onto other side and repeat with other arm.

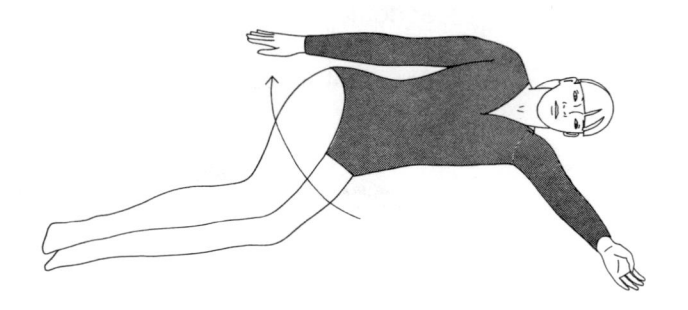

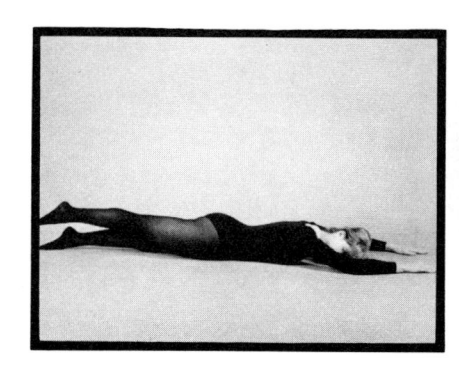

12 Prone Pelvic Rock with Lifts

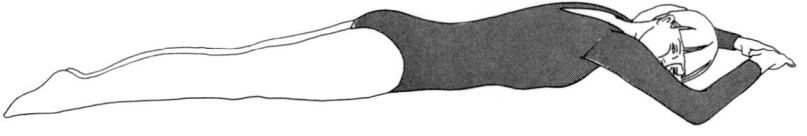

1 Lie flat on stomach on mat, head resting on cheek.

2 Tighten buttocks and curl tailbone inward for slight pelvic rock. A space should appear under the lower abdominal area. Hold briefly; release.
Repeat 4 times.

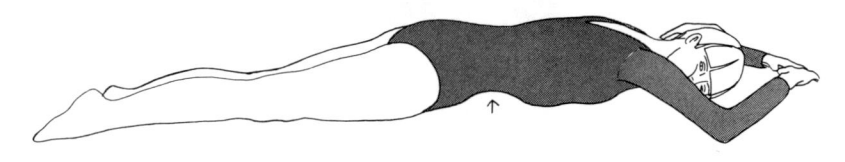

3 Repeat pelvic rock and maintain. Lift right leg very slightly off mat.

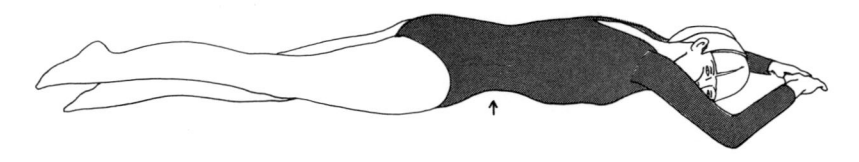

4 Return leg to mat; release rock.
Alternating legs, do 4 lifts with each leg.

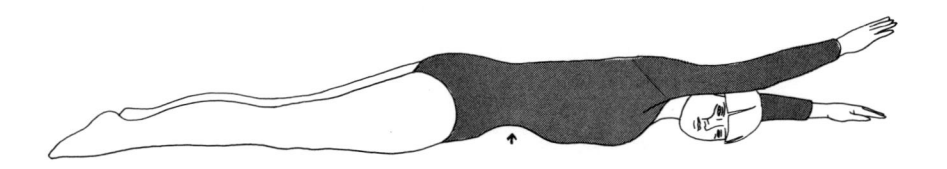

5 Lying in prone position as in position 1, extend arms forward along mat.
Do pelvic rock; lift right arm with elbow straight.

6 Lower arm to mat; release rock.
Alternating arms, do 4 lifts with each arm.

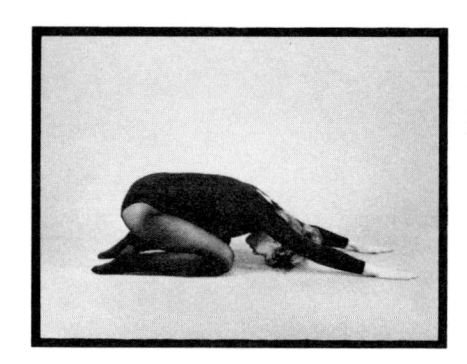

13 Cat Rest

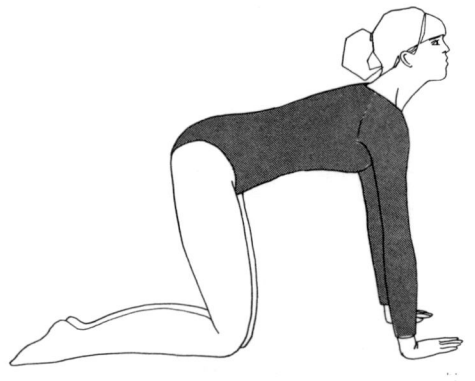

1 Get up on hands and knees, palms under shoulders, knees hip-width apart.

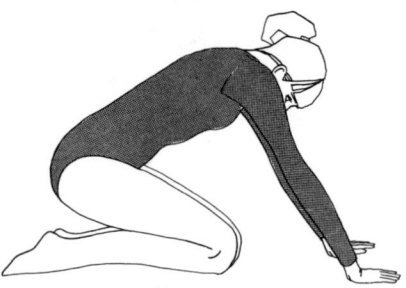

2 Sit back on haunches. Drop head toward chest

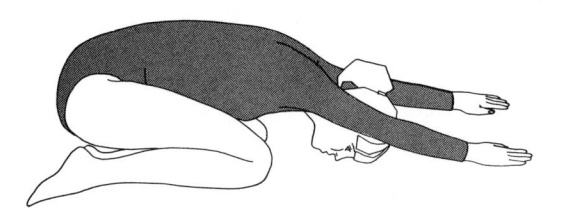

3 slide arms forward until forehead rests on mat.

• **Hold the position until the back, shoulders, and arms feel stretched out and rested. The Cat Rest can be done at any time in the series when you feel the need of a stretch-out.**

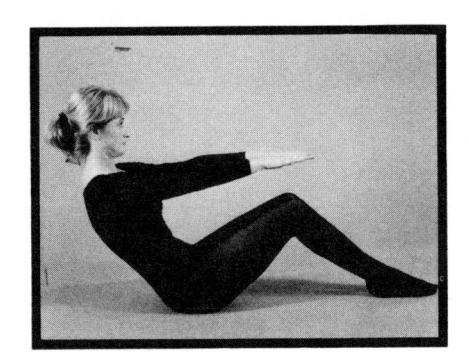

14
Sit-Back

1 Sit on mat, knees up, feet flat and comfortably apart.

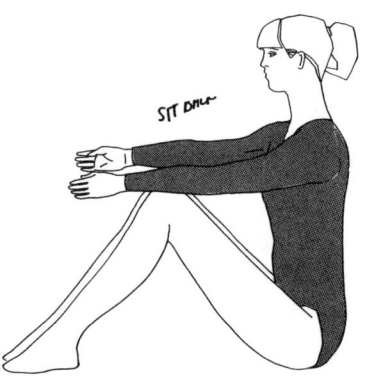

2 Raise arms straight out in front at shoulder level; be sure to keep your spine straight.

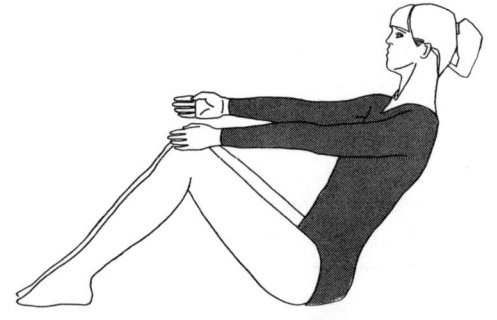

3 Using the abdominal muscles, lean back to a slow count of 4 until upper body is at 45-degree angle to legs. Hold for slow count of 4.

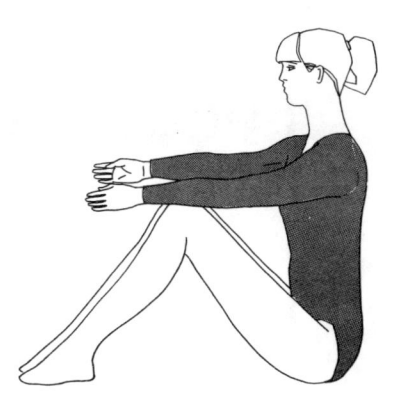

4 To slow count of 4 return to upright sitting position.
Repeat 4 times at start. Repeats are less important than correct performance each time.

- **If you can't get back to 45 degrees at the start, get back only as far as you can. The object is to work the abdominals. If you cannot hold the sit-back angle and have to shift, bend, or struggle to sit up again, you're going too far for your present capacity. Slow, persistent, and correct performance is more important than wide angle.**
- **Concentrate on the abdominal muscles and on keeping your back straight, but don't allow the spine to stiffen.**

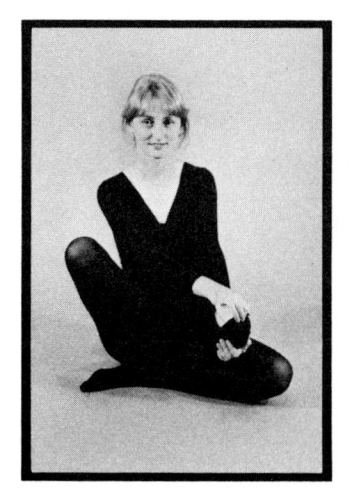

15
Foot Reviver

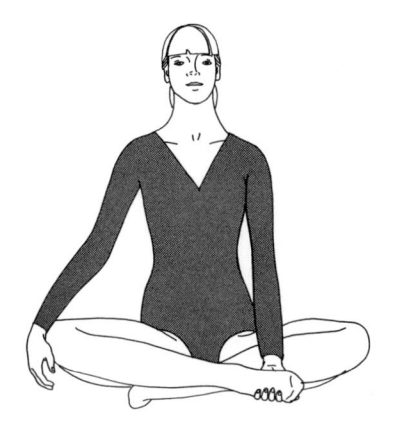

1 Sit loosely cross-legged, body upright, holding right foot in left hand.

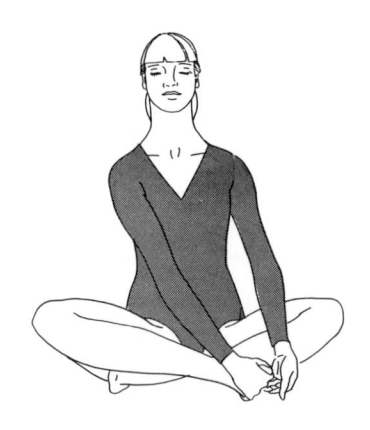

2 Using fingers of both hands, pull toes of right foot apart, trying for as much distance as possible.

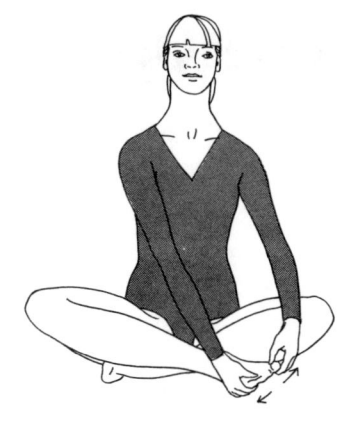

3 Using fingers of right hand, gently rotate toes, one at a time. Work gently—foot bones are tiny and fragile.

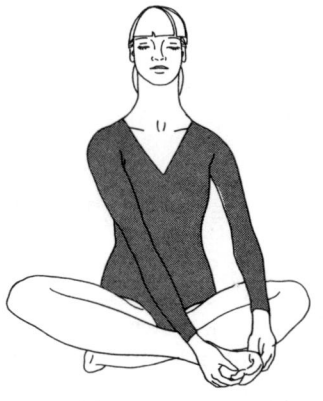

4 With right hand, press toes of right foot down into clenched position, then relax.

5 Shift position and repeat with left foot.

6 Stretch legs out forward; try to spread toes apart without using hands.

- **This foot massage is an amazing restorative for tired or cramped feet at any time, but if you do it in the morning before even getting out of bed, you'll find that your loosened and more mobile foot bones will tire much less easily.**

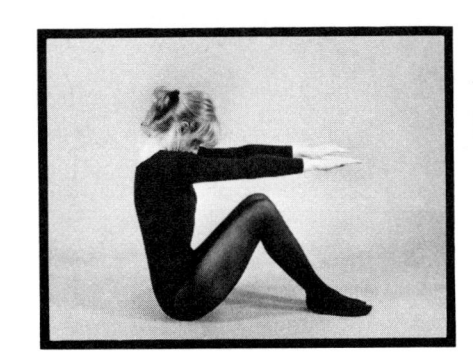

16 Curl-Up

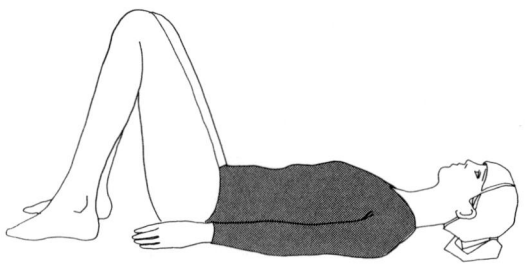

1 Lie on back in tent position, arms at sides. Pull small of back down into mat; tighten buttocks to curl up tailbone.

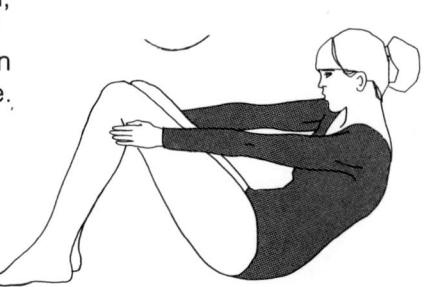

2 Maintaining the curl, raise the head, bringing chin in close to neck. Reach hands toward knees.

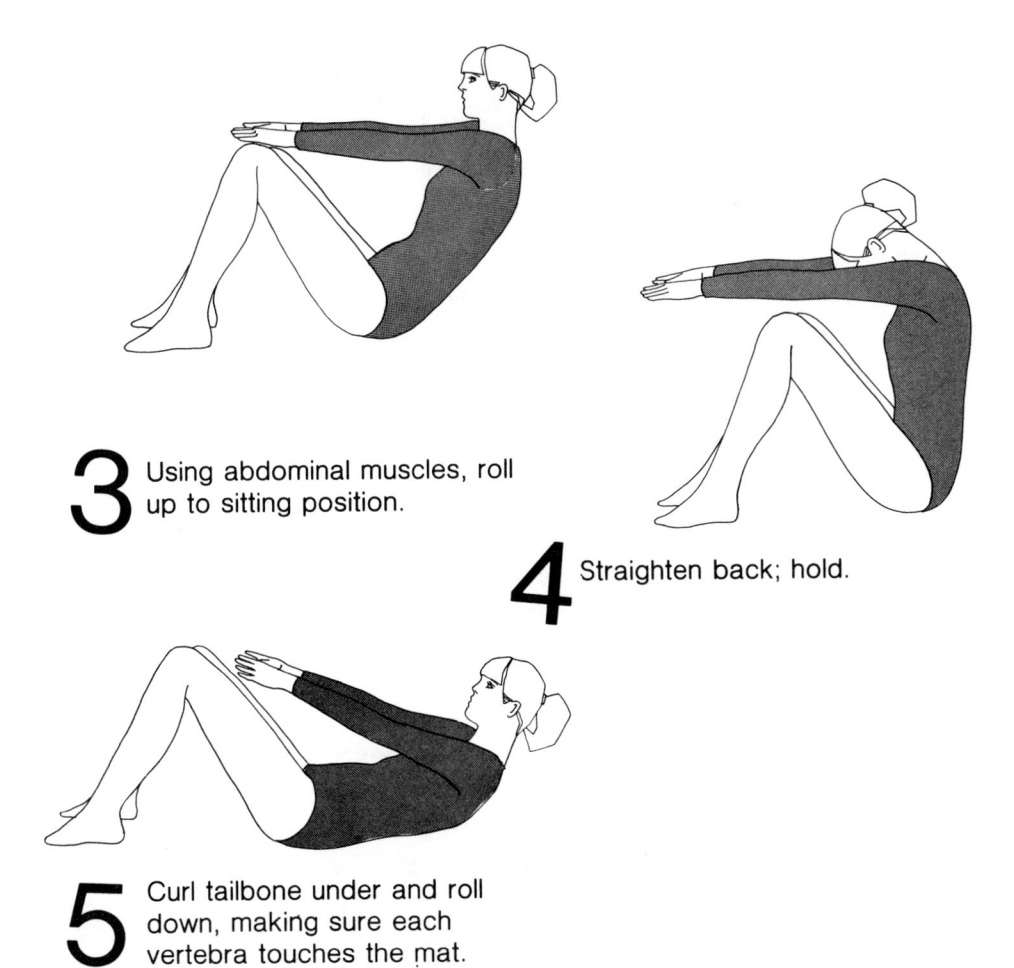

3 Using abdominal muscles, roll up to sitting position.

4 Straighten back; hold.

5 Curl tailbone under and roll down, making sure each vertebra touches the mat.

Repeat 4 times at start. As strength improves, increase to 8 times.

- **Between curl-ups, lie relaxed, breathing normally.**
- **Don't use arms or shoulders to power the sit-up. Power should come from the abdominals, and will increase with practice.**
- **As in all exercises calling for roll-down, be sure each section of the spine can be felt rolling down on the mat, from bottom to top.**

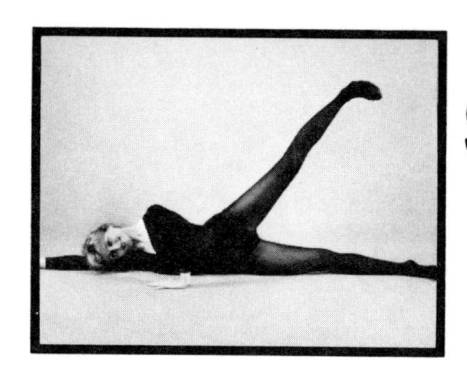

17 Side Leg Lift

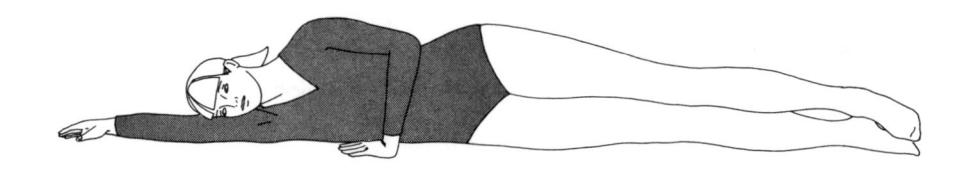

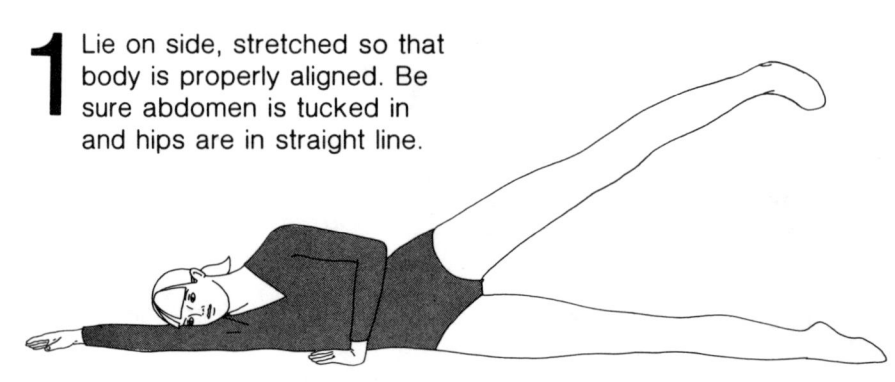

1 Lie on side, stretched so that body is properly aligned. Be sure abdomen is tucked in and hips are in straight line.

2 With knee and foot turned slightly inward, lift the top leg as high as it will easily go. The movement is from the hip.

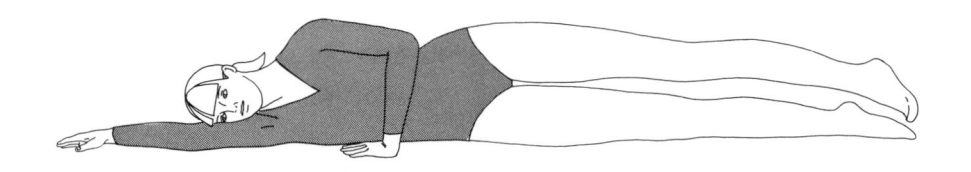

3 Lower the leg to within an inch or so of the bottom leg, but do not allow them to touch.

Repeat 8 times, then shift to other side and repeat with other leg.

- **Both legs should remain straight throughout, but not locked.**
- **Maintain the tucked-in position of the abdomen, the pulled-back small of the back, and the head and shoulders in good alignment. Don't allow the hips to shift.**

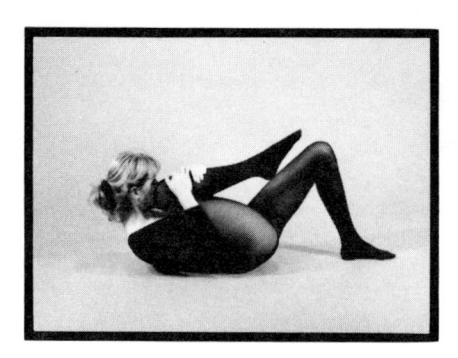

18 Knee Kiss

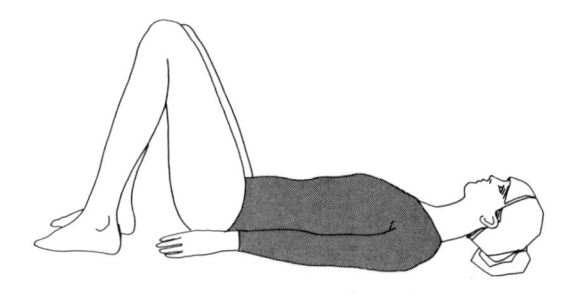

1 Lie on back in tent position, arms at sides.

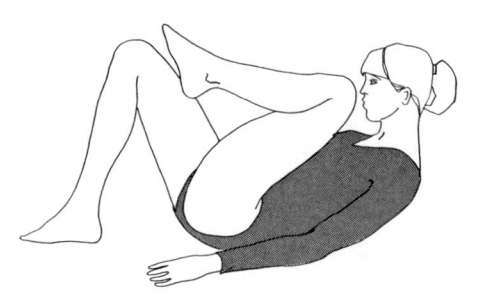

2 Bring one knee up to chest. Simultaneously roll up head to bring forehead as close to knee as possible.

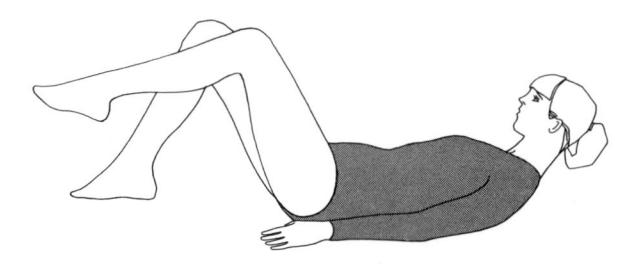

3 Roll down head, return knee to position 1.
Alternating legs, do 4 kisses with each leg.

• **Keep the small of the back pulled in to the mat throughout.**

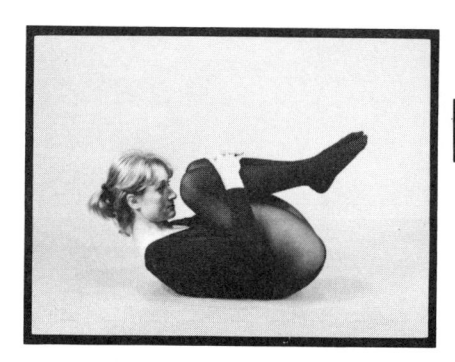

19 Body Curl

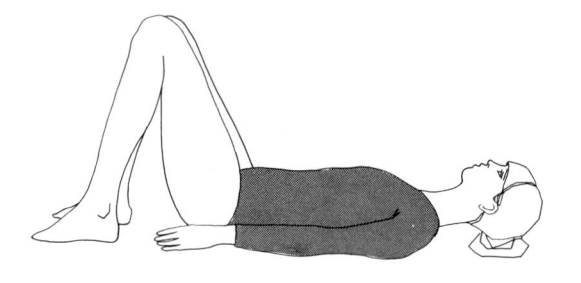

1 Lie on back in tent position.

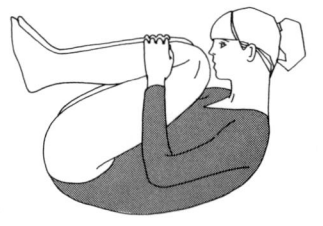

2 Roll up; clasp hands around knees, pulling them in toward body.

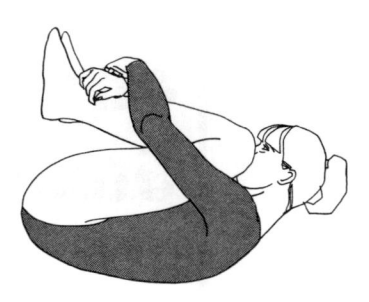

3 Drop head toward chest, pull hard on knees, and curl body in upon itself. Hold.

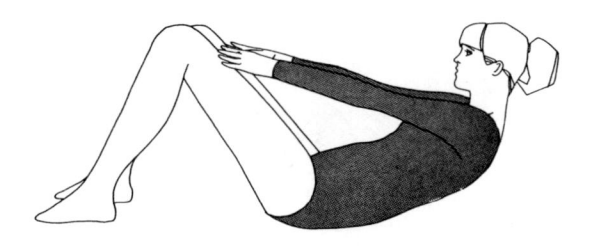

4 Release tension and unclasp arms; roll down slowly, controlling so that each vertebra from bottom to top touches the mat in turn.

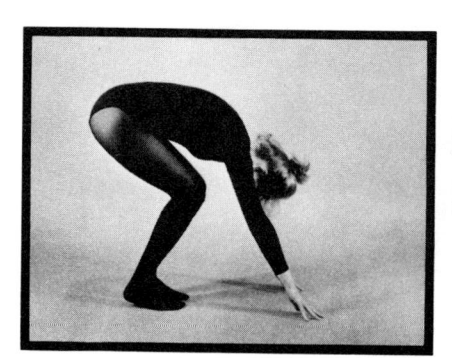

20 Stretching Stand-Up

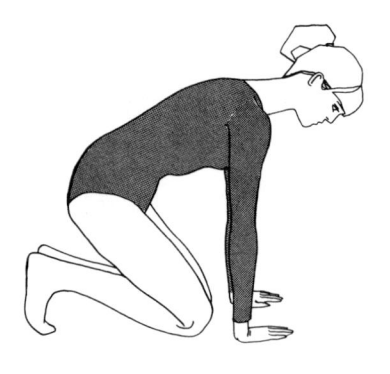

1 Get down on hands and knees. Tuck toes under so that they bend up toward front of legs.

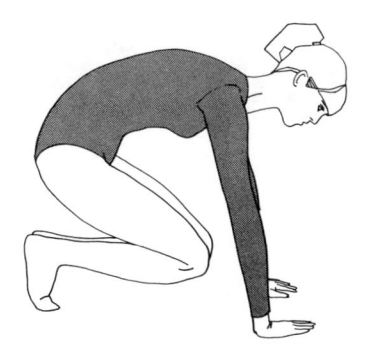

2 Curve back up and push back onto feet. Stand up, coming into good-posture position.

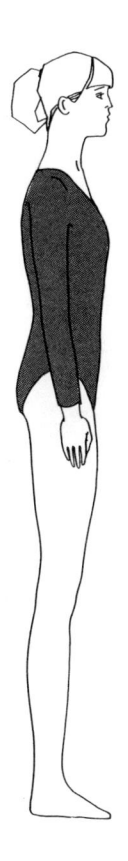

- You can simply stand up, of course, but doing it this way provides an extra stretch for the back and some helpful flexing for the toes. It's a good habit to get into.

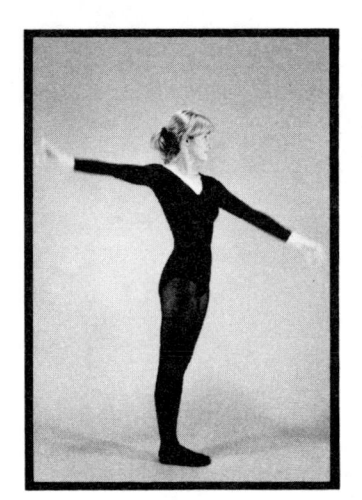

21 Arm Swing

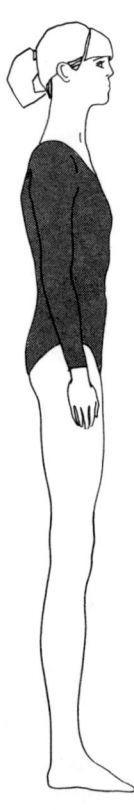

1 Stand with arms loose at sides; check posture. Swing right arm fully around, up over head like a paddle wheel.

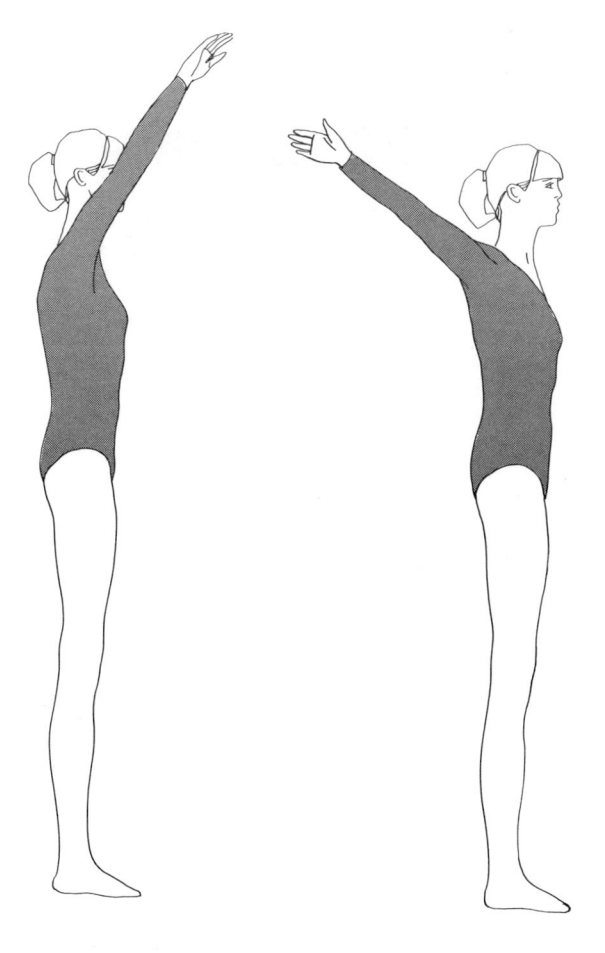

2 Swing right arm fully around, up over head like a paddle wheel.

Finish with arm at side. Repeat 8 times in each direction with each arm. Repeat 8 times in each direction with both arms.

- **Maintain good posture throughout.**
- **Keeping the head straight may tighten the neck. A few head rolls at the end of the exercise will release any tension there.**

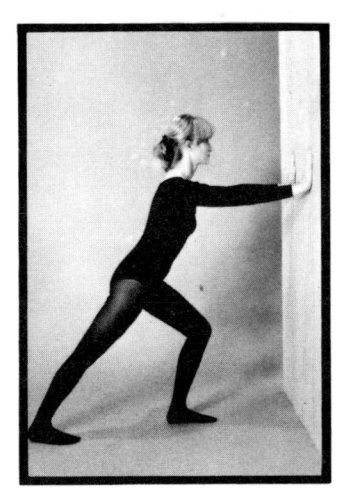

22 Standing Hamstring Stretch

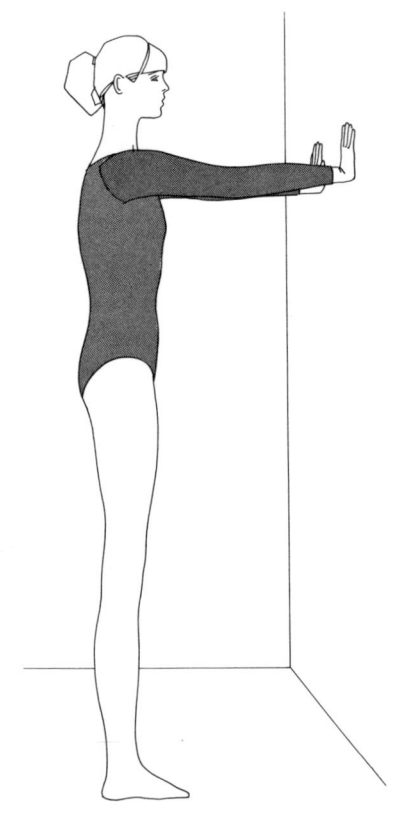

1 Stand about 2 feet away from wall, facing it, feet parallel and comfortably apart. Place palms flat against wall just under shoulder level.

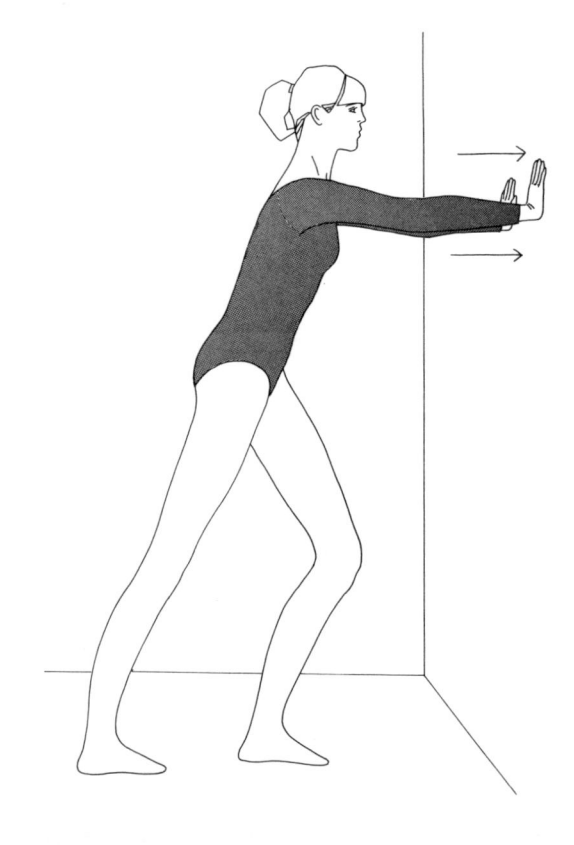

2 Thrust back with right leg, keeping right foot flat on floor if possible, simultaneously bending left knee.

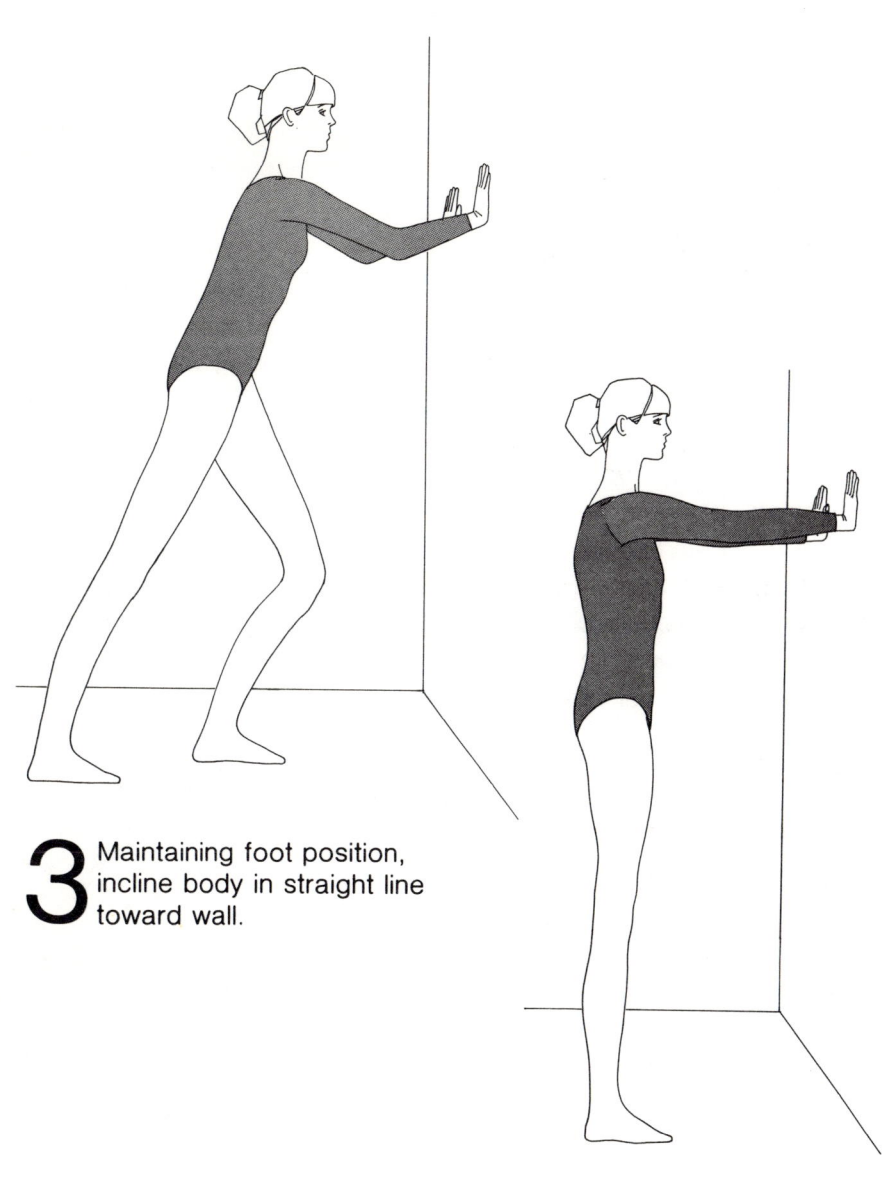

3 Maintaining foot position, incline body in straight line toward wall.

4 Hold; push body upright and return feet to parallel position.
Repeat with left leg.

A Last Word

When you opened this book, chances are your body was in need of attention.

Now you have worked your way to this end page. Hopefully, on the way, you discovered a new world of physical well being.

So far, you have done your part, just as we have. We can't do more. You can. Exercise is like dieting. It works only if you stay with it. Make exercise as basic a part of your daily existence as brushing your teeth, going to work, eating, sleeping. You will have the time of your life, all your life.

Elaine Quinn